The Castor Oil Bible Unveiled

The Ultimate Guide to Unleashing the Power of Nature's Remedy/ 200+ Recipes for Your Well-being, Health and Beauty (Nature's Elixir for Modern Wellness)

Lizzy Moore

COPYRIGHT © 2024- All Right Reserved

NOELLE BOWMAN

Disclaimer Notice:

Please note the information contained within this document is for educational and entertainment purposes only. All effort has been executed to present accurate, up-to-date, and reliable, complete information. No warranties of any kind are declared or implied. Readers acknowledge that the author is not engaging in the rendering of legal, financial, medical or professional advice. The content within this book has been derived from various sources. Please consult a licensed professional before attempting any techniques outlined in this book.
By reading this document, the reader agrees that under no circumstances is the author responsible for any losses, direct or indirect, which are incurred as a result of the use of information contained within this document, including, but not limited to, -errors, omissions, or inaccuracies.

Table of Contents

CHAPTER 1

INTRODUCTION

Castor Oil: Its Historical Significance and Cultural Impact

Castor oil, derived from the seeds of the castor plant, has played a pivotal role in various industries, marking its importance as one of the world's key industrial oils since ancient times. These seeds have been discovered in ancient Egyptian burial sites dating back to 4000 B.C. The Ebers Papyrus, an ancient Egyptian medical document from 1500 B.C., mentions its use to shield eyes from irritations. Historically, castor oil was incorporated into facial oils and used in lamps for lighting. In the United States, it has long been utilized for its medicinal properties, dating back to pioneer days. In the late 1800s, itinerant salesmen marketed castor oil, often diluted with alcohol, as a remedy for ailments ranging from constipation to heartburn and as a labor inducer. Currently, it is employed both as a laxative and topically in the form of packs or poultices.

The castor plant, or Ricinus communis, originates from the Ethiopian region of East Africa but is now prevalent in warm and tropical climates globally, often becoming invasive in regions like the southwestern U.S. These plants thrive in well-drained, nutrient-rich soils in areas with ample sunlight, heat, and moisture, growing 6–15 feet tall within a single season. The plant exhibits unique foliage, with large leaves that can span 4–30 inches, and features distinct flowers with separate male and female parts that bloom almost year-round. The seeds are known for their strong ejecting mechanism when mature and their unique, intricately patterned shells.

The plant received its name "castor" from English traders who confused its oil with that of another plant, Vitex agnus-castus, while the genus name Ricinus, meaning "tick" in Latin, was inspired by the seed's resemblance to a blood-engorged tick, as noted by the Swedish botanist Carolus Linnaeus.

Despite its rapid growth and striking appearance, the cultivation of the castor plant is discouraged due to the high toxicity of its seeds, which contain ricin, a potent toxin. It is critical, especially in areas where the plant grows wild, to educate children to recognize and avoid the castor plant and its seeds. The plant's toxic potential is so significant that even a minuscule amount of ricin can be fatal if ingested or entered into the bloodstream through wounds.

Recently, ricin has been spotlighted due to its potential use in terrorism, though it is more commonly employed in targeted assassination attempts. The CDC classifies it as a B-list bioterrorism agent due to its ease of production and moderate threat level. However, research is also exploring ricin's application in cancer treatment, particularly in the development of immunotoxins designed to target and destroy tumor cells selectively.

Throughout history, castor oil's influence has spanned across continents and cultures:

1.   Ancient Egypt: Highly valued for its medicinal benefits, used topically for skin conditions and eye irritations.

2.   Ayurveda and Traditional Medicine: Utilized in Ayurvedic practices for its purgative properties and believed to help balance bodily systems and enhance well-being.

3.   Traditional Chinese and Asian Medicine: Employed for its anti-inflammatory and pain-relieving properties, often applied externally to soothe discomfort and inflammation.

The Science Behind Castor Oil: Chemical Composition and Properties

Chemical Composition

•   Ricinoleic Acid: Castor oil is predominantly composed of ricin oleic acid, which accounts for about 90% of its makeup. This unique fatty acid distinguishes castor oil from other vegetable oils and is the secret behind its numerous health benefits.

•   Other Fatty Acids and Triglycerides: Besides ricin oleic acid, castor oil contains oleic acid, linoleic acid, and stearic acid. It also contains triglycerides, which are known to enhance skin hydration and improve the skin's barrier function.

•   Beneficial Properties: The high concentration of ricin oleic acid in castor oil may reduce inflammation and improve blood circulation. It also boosts the immune system and provides protection against bacterial and fungal infections. These properties make castor oil a trusted natural remedy for various health issues.

General Use of Castor Oil

Internal Uses: Castor oil is a potent cathartic or purgative, effective in stimulating both the small and large intestines. It is used to cleanse the bowels post-food poisoning and to alleviate constipation. In medical settings, it is sometimes used to prepare patients for abdominal scans, such as X-rays of the colon or kidneys. Castor oil acts as a stimulant laxative, which increases muscle contractions in the intestines to help move stool through the bowels. While effective, this type of laxative may cause side effects and is typically recommended for short-term use only. For self-treatment, it is important to follow manufacturer's guidelines and drink plenty of fluids to ease stool passage. Castor oil is best taken on an empty stomach for quicker results, and mixing it with cold orange juice can improve its taste. Flavored options are also available.

External Uses: Topically, castor oil is applied to treat common skin conditions like corns, warts, ringworm, abscesses, bruises, dry skin, dermatitis, sunburn, and open sores. It is also found in hair tonics, cosmetics, and contraceptive creams and jellies. To treat corns, castor oil is applied directly to the affected area, which is then covered with felt pads and silk tape to enhance absorption.

Nonmedical Uses: Castor oil and its derivatives find extensive use in various industrial products, such as paints, varnishes, fabric coatings, insulation materials, food containers, soap, ink, plastics, brake fluids, insecticidal oils, and firearms. It is a key raw material in the production of synthetic resins like nylon, and is used in high-performance motor oils for racing cars and motorcycles. Additionally, it serves as a fuel additive for two-cycle engines, enhancing the exhaust's distinct aroma. Despite its unpleasant smell and taste, castor oil is used to synthesize artificial scents and flavors.

Versatile Uses Through the Ages

1.   Digestive Health: Traditionally, castor oil was consumed as a strong laxative to relieve constipation and stimulate bowel movements.

2.   Skin and Hair Care: Its moisturizing properties make it a popular component in skincare and haircare products, promoting wound healing and hair conditioning.

3.   Inducing Labor: Some cultures have used castor oil to induce labor, although this practice is medically debated and should be approached with caution.

4.   Arthritis and Pain Relief: Historically, castor oil has been applied topically to alleviate joint pain and muscle soreness.

5.   Natural Lubricant and Industrial Uses: Due to its high viscosity and stability, castor oil is used as a lubricant in machinery and engines and is incorporated into numerous industrial products.

Modern Applications and Considerations In contemporary settings, castor oil continues to be valued for its role in beauty and wellness products, massage therapies, and occasionally as a laxative. However, its potent effects mean that it should be used with medical oversight, particularly for internal applications. The enduring legacy of castor oil through the ages underscores its adaptability and continued relevance in both traditional and modern contexts, making it a versatile and beneficial oil across various domains.

Types of Castor Oil

Castor oil comes in various forms, each with unique extraction methods and uses:

•   Yellow Castor Oil: This type is also known as cold-pressed castor oil. It is extracted from castor seeds at temperatures below 49°C (120°F) and refined without heat or chemicals to preserve its natural properties. Yellow castor oil is commonly used for its cosmetic and medicinal benefits due to its high purity and nutrient content.

- Black Castor Oil: Known alternatively as Jamaican or African black castor oil, this variety is produced by pressing roasted castor seeds, which imparts a dark brown or black color and a distinct aroma. The roasting process is believed to enhance the oil's effectiveness, particularly in promoting hair health.

Castor oil is renowned for its potency and backed by some research for its health effects. Further details on its uses and benefits will be discussed as you continue reading.

CHAPTER 2

Understanding Castor oil

How To Make A Castor Oil Pack

A castor oil pack can be an effective remedy for various ailments. Here's a simple guide on how to prepare one:

What You Need:

- Pure hexane-free castor oil

- 1 large glass jar with a lid

- Dye-free wool, unbleached

Directions:

1. Fold the dye-free wool cloth into three layers.

2. Place the folded wool into the glass jar and pour enough castor oil over it to saturate. Seal the jar and shake well to ensure the oil is evenly distributed throughout the cloth.

3. When needed, remove the wool cloth from the jar for use as your castor oil pack.

Application: Before applying the pack, lay out some old towels where you will be lying down. Place the saturated wool cloth on the affected area of your body, cover it with plastic wrap, and elevate your feet slightly. Relax in this position for 20 to 30 minutes to allow the oil to absorb into the skin. Afterwards, use a clean, dry cloth to wipe off any excess oil.

Side Effects of Castor Oil

Serious Side Effects:

- Skin rash

- Weakness or tiredness

- Confusion

- Irregular heartbeat

- Muscle aches

Less Serious Side Effects:

- Diarrhea or cramps

- Burping

- Nausea

Instructions for Using a Castor Oil Pack

Preparation and Use:

1.   Place the required amount of castor oil (typically 1 tablespoon per use) in a jar or on a large old towel.

2.   If using a jar or glass container, store the saturated material in the refrigerator or a cool, dark place to prevent it from going rancid.

3.   Position the castor oil pack on desired areas, such as the mid-section or directly over specific organs like the liver, gallbladder, or thyroid.

4.   Place a hot water bottle or heating pad over the pack, using an old towel or pillowcase as a barrier to protect from oil stains.

5.   Relax with the pack in place, ideally for an hour with legs elevated. If the pack is designed to be worn, you can continue your day or sleep with it on.

6.   After removing the pack, either rub in the excess oil or clean it off depending on your next activities.

7.   Store the used pack appropriately and wash any other used textiles separately. Avoid machine washing the actual castor oil pack.

Frequency of Use:

- For optimal results, use the castor oil pack at least four times a week for one month. Daily use is reported to yield the best benefits.

- For ongoing maintenance, using the pack once a week or a few times a month can help manage or prevent recurring issues.

• The pack can be reused several times (up to 2-3 months), adding more oil as needed to keep it saturated.

Note: If you experience stomach upset or other discomforts, consider taking a break or reducing the frequency of use. Adjust the routine to what feels best for your body, and always consult a healthcare professional if unsure about its use, especially if dealing with serious health issues.

Nutritional Value of Castor Oil

Castor oil is unique in its composition, with ricin oleic acid making up about 90% of its fatty acid content. This acid is beneficial for the skin, helping to treat conditions like dermatitis, psoriasis, and acne. It also aids digestion when broken down in the small intestine. Other components of castor oil include:

• Oleic acid (6%-2%)

• Linoleic acid (5%-2%)

• Dihydroxy stearic acid (0.5%-0.3%)

• High quantities of Vitamin E and Omega 6 and 9 fatty acids, which support cell longevity, energy provision, and inflammation reduction.

CHAPTER 3

Identifying and Finding Quality Castor Oil

Selecting high-quality castor oil is crucial for maximizing its therapeutic benefits. Look for cold-pressed or expeller-pressed varieties, which preserve the nutrients without high heat or chemicals. Opting for organic and hexane-free castor oil ensures lower exposure to potentially harmful substances. Quality castor oil is available at health food stores, online platforms, and shops specializing in natural products.

How to Take Castor Oil

Follow these guidelines for safe consumption:

•	Adhere to dosage instructions provided by your doctor or as stated on the label.

•	Consume on an empty stomach to enhance effectiveness.

•	Stay hydrated by drinking 6 to 8 glasses of water daily.

•	Use the proper method to take the oil, whether it's swallowing capsules whole or dissolving granules in liquid.

What to Do If You Miss a Dose of Castor Oil

If you miss a dose, take it as soon as possible, unless it's near the time for your next dose. In that case, skip the missed dose and continue with your regular schedule. Do not double up doses.

Contraindications for Castor Oil Use

Avoid castor oil if you have allergies to stimulant laxatives, intestinal blockages, symptoms of appendicitis, or unexplained rectal bleeding. Always consult with a healthcare provider before starting any new treatment.

Castor Oil Warnings

When using castor oil, consider the following precautions:

- **Medical Conditions**: Inform your doctor if you are pregnant, breastfeeding, or if you have diabetes, high blood pressure, or heart disease.

- **Children's Use**: Do not give laxatives to children under 6 years old without consulting a doctor.

- **Duration of Use**: Avoid using this laxative for more than 1 week unless specifically directed by your doctor. Prolonged use can lead to dependency and might damage your bowels.

- **Potential Symptoms**: Be aware of possible symptoms such as skin rash or general weakness and fatigue.

Castor Oil Interactions

Castor oil should be used cautiously with other medications due to possible interactions:

- **Timing with Medications**: Do not use a laxative within 2 hours of taking other medications.

- **Specific Interactions**: Avoid using a laxative containing bisacodyl, such as Dulcolax, within 1 hour before or after consuming milk or taking antacids.

CHAPTER 4

RECIPES: Natural Castor Oil Recipes for Hair Care

Castor Oil Formula for Reducing Grey Hair

Castor and Coconut Oil Mixture for Early Grey Hair

For ages, coconut oil has been a staple in Indian hair care, thanks to its lauric acid content, which easily penetrates the hair shaft.

Ingredients

- ½ teaspoon of Castor Oil

- 1 teaspoon of Coconut Oil

- 3-4 drops of Lavender Oil

How to Prepare the Oil Mixture

1.   In a small bowl, combine all oils.

2.   Shake the mixture gently to ensure the oils blend well, despite their different densities.

3.   Mix thoroughly to create a deep conditioning mask aimed at promoting hair growth.

Application Instructions

1.   Gently massage the oil mixture into your scalp, working it through to the tips of your hair.

2.   Gather your hair into a bun and let the oil sit for at least one hour.

3.   Wash out the oil using your regular shampoo, repeating the process to ensure all oil is removed due to the thickness of castor oil.

Castor and Mustard Oil for Hair Revitalization

This combination rejuvenates the scalp and restores shine to your hair.

Ingredients

- 3 tablespoons of Castor Oil
- 1 tablespoon of Mustard Oil

How to Prepare

- Combine both oils in a bowl.

Application Instructions

1. Massage the mixture into your hair and scalp for ten minutes to stimulate circulation.

2. Wash your hair after about an hour.

Castor and Amla Oil for Darkening Hair

Ideal for thinning or lifeless hair, this intensive overnight mask hydrates the scalp and helps combat premature greying.

Ingredients

- 5 tablespoons of Castor Oil
- 2 tablespoons of Amla Oil

How to Prepare

- Blend the oils in a mixing bowl.

Application Instructions

1. Evenly apply the oil mixture to your hair.

2. Massage your scalp gently, then cover your head with a scarf or shower cap overnight.

3. Wash and condition your hair the following morning.

Castor Oil for Eyelash and Eyebrow Growth

Castor Oil with Olive Oil for Healthy Nails & Cuticles

Healthy hands are a reflection of a well-maintained body, and Castor Oil is perfect for nourishing nails and cuticles.

Ingredients

- 10 drops of Castor Oil
- 10 drops of Virgin Olive Oil

Directions

1. Remove any nail polish and file your nails to the desired shape.
2. Clean your hands to eliminate any dead skin.
3. Apply a blend of olive and castor oil to your cuticles with a cotton pad.
4. Massage the oils into your nails and cuticles for 2-3 minutes.
5. Let the oil absorb overnight.

Castor Oil and Coconut Oil for Eyelashes

A nourishing blend to enhance the appearance and health of your eyelashes.

Ingredients

- 5-7 ml of Castor Oil
- 2 drops of Virgin Coconut Oil
- ½ tablespoon of Petroleum Jelly

Directions

1. Mix the oils and petroleum jelly in a small bottle.
2. Apply gently to your eyelashes using a cotton ball.
3. Wash off after 4 hours. Repeat twice a week for best results.

Castor Oil and Vitamin E for Eyelashes

Promotes thick, healthy eyelashes by protecting them from environmental stresses.

Ingredients

- 8 ml of Castor Oil

- 2 drops of Vitamin E Oil

Directions

1. Combine the oils in a small container.

2. Apply to your eyelashes with a clean mascara stick.

3. Rinse with water after 6 hours.

4. For optimal results, repeat this process twice a week.

Castor Oil and Rosemary Oil for Eyelash Enhancement

This combination is perfect for enhancing eyelash thickness due to castor oil's rich vitamin and mineral content and rosemary oil's ability to improve circulation.

Ingredients

- 5 ml of Castor Oil

- 3 drops of Rosemary Essential Oil

Directions

1. Combine the castor oil and rosemary oil in a bowl and mix thoroughly.

2. Carefully apply the mixture to your lashes with a clean mascara wand.

3. Leave the solution on overnight, or for a minimum of 6 hours.

4. Wash it off with running water. Use this treatment weekly.

Castor Oil and Olive Oil for Eyelashes

Rich in vitamins A and E, olive oil, combined with castor oil, provides dual benefits for eyelash health.

Ingredients

- 10 ml of Castor Oil

- 3 drops of Virgin Olive Oil

Directions

1. Mix the castor oil and olive oil and let it sit for 5 minutes.

2. Use a cotton stick to apply the oil blend to your eyelashes.

3. After 4 hours, wash the oil off with water.

4. For best results, apply this blend weekly at night.

Castor Oil and Almond Oil for Eyelashes

Almond oil is loaded with Vitamin E, magnesium, and essential lipids, making it an excellent partner to castor oil for promoting lush, healthy eyelashes.

Ingredients

- 8 ml of Castor Oil

- 2 drops of Sweet Almond Oil

Directions

1. Mix the oils well in a small container.

2. Apply the mixture to both upper and lower lashes using a mascara wand.

3. Allow it to sit overnight, or for at least 6 hours.

4. Clean it off with water or soft wipes. Apply this blend once every 15 days.

Castor Oil and Vitamin E Oil for Eyebrow Growth

Boost your eyebrow care with this enriched castor oil and vitamin E blend.

Ingredients

- 10 drops of Castor Oil
- 6 drops of Vitamin E oil

Directions

1. In a bowl, combine the castor oil and vitamin E oil until smooth.
2. Apply to your eyebrows using a q-tip.
3. Let the mixture sit for 24 hours.
4. Wash off with lukewarm water or a gentle hair cleanser.

Vitamin E Oil, Castor Oil, and Coconut Oil for Eyebrow Growth

A hydrating blend suitable for nourishing and enhancing eyebrows.

Ingredients

- 10 drops of Castor Oil
- 4 drops of Vitamin E Oil
- 5 drops of Virgin Coconut Oil

Directions

1. Start by pouring the coconut oil into a small container.
2. Add the castor oil and vitamin E oil, mixing until creamy.
3. Use a q-tip to apply this mixture to your eyebrows.
4. Leave the mixture on overnight.
5. Rinse your eyebrows with warm water or herbal shampoo.

Onion Juice and Castor Oil for Eyebrow Growth

Combining onion juice's high sulfur content with castor oil can significantly boost eyebrow growth.

Ingredients

- 10 Drops of Castor Oil

- 2 tablespoons of Onion Juice

Directions

Directions

1. Mix the castor oil and onion juice in a small bowl.

2. Apply the mixture to your eyebrows and massage gently in a circular motion for 5-8 minutes.

3. Let it sit for 15-20 minutes.

4. Rinse off with lukewarm water or a bit of herbal shampoo.

Castor Oil Eyelash Serum

Castor Oil is excellent for strengthening eyelash strands and preventing fall-out. It hydrates lashes and serves as a cost-effective alternative to commercial eyelash lengthening products. Regular application, combined with a balanced diet, can lead to longer, thicker lashes, potentially eliminating the need for mascara.

Ingredients

- ½ teaspoon Castor Oil

- ¼ teaspoon Vitamin E

- ¼ teaspoon Almond Oil

Procedure

1. Combine these essential oils in an amber-colored glass bottle.

2. Use a clean mascara wand to apply the oil mixture to your lashes.

3.   Apply daily to notice improvements in lash length and thickness.

4.   Optionally, apply at night and leave on overnight for intensive treatment.

Nature Castor Oil for Deep Conditioning and Scalp Treatment

Rosemary Hair Growth Serum

Rosemary essential oil is celebrated for its hair growth properties and its ability to address dandruff and scalp itching.

Ingredients

- 6 drops Rosemary Essential Oil

- 1 tablespoon Castor Oil

- 1 tablespoon Argan Oil or Jojoba Oil

- 1 oz Dropper Bottle

Directions

1.   Combine all ingredients in the dropper bottle.

2.   Shake well to blend.

3.   Apply a few drops to your fingertips and smooth the oil over your hair, from mid-length to ends, on either wet or dry hair.

4.   Alternatively, use as a weekly scalp massage oil.

Homemade Castor Oil Hydrating Shampoo

Prepare your own hydrating shampoo with castor oil for enhanced hair health.

Ingredients

- A can of Coconut Milk

- 1 tablespoon Castor Oil
- 1 tablespoon Jojoba Oil
- 1 tablespoon Essential Oil of choice
- 2 tablespoons Organic Honey
- 2 tablespoons Apple Cider Vinegar

Directions

1.   Mix all ingredients in a bowl until smooth.

2.   Take a quarter of the mixture and massage it into your scalp with circular motions.

3.   Leave on for 3 to 5 minutes, then rinse off.

Castor Oil Hair Mask for a Healthy Scalp

This simple hair mask uses castor oil to improve scalp and hair health.

Ingredients

- Castor Oil
- Coconut Oil

Directions

1.   Mix a few drops of castor oil with half a cup of coconut oil.

2.   Stir well to combine thoroughly.

3.   Apply to your hair before bedtime and leave it overnight.

4.   For best results, use this method twice a week.

Healthy Scalp Treatment Oil

This treatment is perfect for dealing with dandruff, dry scalp, and flakiness.

Ingredients

- 1 drop Tea Tree Oil

- 1 drop Lavender Essential Oil

- 1 tablespoon Castor Oil

- 1 tablespoon Virgin Coconut Oil

Directions

1. Combine castor oil and coconut oil in a glass bowl.

2. Warm the mixture in a double boiler to a comfortable temperature.

3. Add the essential oils once warm.

4. Apply the warm oil to your scalp and massage gently.

5. Leave on for 30 minutes to an hour, or overnight if preferred.

6. Wash out with your regular shampoo and conditioner.

Simple Hair Growth Serum

This easy-to-make serum uses a blend of oils known for promoting hair growth.

Ingredients

- 3 Tablespoons of Castor Oil

- 1 Tablespoon of Jojoba Oil or Argan Oil

- 2 oz glass bottle with glass dropper

Directions

1. Blend the oils until smooth and transfer to the 2 oz glass bottle.

2. Apply a few drops to the scalp and massage gently for 5 minutes.

Complex Hair Growth Serum

A more robust serum featuring a mix of nourishing oils for an extra boost in hair health and growth.

Ingredients

- 2 teaspoons of Castor Oil
- 2 teaspoons of Almond Oil
- 2 teaspoons of Coconut Oil
- 2 teaspoons of Olive Oil
- 2-3 drops of Lavender Essential Oil
- 1 Tablespoon of Aloe Vera Juice (optional)

Directions

1. Combine all ingredients until smooth.
2. Store in a 2 oz glass bottle.
3. Apply a few drops to the scalp and massage for 5 minutes.

Coconut Oil Hair Mask

Ideal for deep conditioning, this mask combines coconut and castor oils for overnight hair nourishment.

Ingredients

- 2 Tablespoons of Castor Oil
- 2 Tablespoons of Coconut Oil

Directions

1. Mix the oils together in a bowl.
2. Heat the mixture in a double boiler until warm.
3. Apply the warm oil to your scalp and hair, massaging gently.
4. Leave it on overnight.
5. Wash your hair in the morning with a mild shampoo.

Jamaican Black Castor Oil Hair Thickening Mask

This potent hair mask uses Jamaican Black Castor Oil and Coconut Oil to protect hair from chemical damage while promoting thickness and health.

Ingredients

- 2 Tablespoons of Jamaican Black Castor Oil

- 2 Tablespoons of Coconut Oil

Directions

1. Mix the oils together in a bowl.

2. Massage the blend into your scalp and hair for about five minutes.

3. Ensure coverage from roots to ends.

4. Cover with a shower cap or towel.

5. Leave on for two hours or overnight.

6. Rinse with lukewarm water and shampoo.

7. Use twice a week for two months to see visible hair growth improvements.

Hibiscus and Castor Oil Hair Growth Recipe

Combining the strengthening properties of onion juice with the shine-enhancing qualities of hibiscus oil, this hair mask promotes fuller and healthier hair.

Ingredients

- 2 Tablespoons of Castor Oil

- 2 Tablespoons of Onion Juice

- 4-5 Drops of Hibiscus Essential Oil

Directions

1. Mix the castor oil and onion juice in a bowl.

2.   Stir in the hibiscus essential oil until well combined.

3.   Apply the blend to your scalp and hair.

4.   Massage gently and leave on for about two hours.

5.   Rinse with lukewarm water and shampoo.

Organic Shea Butter Coconut Oil and Castor Oil Mix

This mix is designed to promote hair growth and moisturize the skin.

Ingredients

- 1/2 Cup Organic Shea Butter

- 2 Tablespoons Fractionated Coconut Oil

- 2-6 Teaspoons Organic Castor Oil

- 7 Drops Rosemary Essential Oil

- 5 Drops Lemongrass Essential Oil

Method

1.   If the Organic Shea Butter is hard, soften it by placing the jar in a bowl of hot water.

2.   Once softened, whip it with a hand mixer for about 30 seconds to make it creamier.

3.   Add the coconut oil and whip for about 10 seconds.

4.   Scrape the sides of the bowl with a plastic spatula.

5.   Add the Organic Castor Oil and essential oils, then whip again for a minute or two until fully incorporated.

6.   Transfer the mix into a sterilized mason jar or container.

7.   Store in a clean, dry place away from water and other contaminants.

Organic Castor Hot Oil Hair Treatment

This treatment uses a blend of organic oils to improve hair strength and texture.

Ingredients

- 30ml Organic Castor Oil

- 30g Organic Virgin Coconut Oil

- 20ml Organic Argan Oil

- 20ml Organic Extra Virgin Olive Oil

- 1ml Organic Rosemary Oil (approx. 20 drops)

Directions

1.	Combine all the carrier oils in a bowl and gently heat in the microwave until the coconut oil melts.

2.	Add the Rosemary oil and stir well.

3.	Check the oil's temperature to ensure it's not too hot before application.

4.	Apply the warm oil to damp hair, coating from root to tip.

5.	Cover your hair with an old towel or t-shirt and leave for 30 minutes to an hour.

6.	Shampoo and condition your hair, possibly shampooing twice to remove all oil.

7.	Allow your hair to air dry.

8.	Store any remaining oil in a dark colored bottle for future treatments. Repeat weekly for best results.

Conditioning Hair Mask

This all-natural hair mask is perfect for restoring moisture to both scalp and hair.

Ingredients

- 2 tbsp Castor Oil
- 1 tbsp Glycerin
- 1 tbsp Apple Cider Vinegar
- 3 beaten eggs

Procedure

1. Combine all ingredients in a bowl and apply to dry hair.
2. Cover hair thoroughly from roots to tips.
3. Wrap with plastic wrap or a shower cap, then cover with a towel.
4. Let the mask sit for 2 hours.
5. Rinse thoroughly with water, using shampoo if necessary.

Thick and Resilient Hair Growth Blend

A simple oil mix that promotes thicker and stronger hair strands.

Ingredients

- Equal parts Castor Oil and Jojoba or Argan Oil

Procedure

1. Mix the oils in a small amber glass bottle.
2. Apply a few drops to the scalp and hair, massaging gently.
3. Use this treatment at night 2-4 times a week for best results.

Castor Oil Hair Mask

This mask uses the nourishing properties of castor and coconut oils for softer, smoother hair.

Ingredients

- ½ Castor Oil

- ½ Coconut Oil

Procedure

1. Blend the oils in a bowl.

2. Gently heat the mixture for 30 seconds, avoiding direct heat and boiling.

3. Massage the warm oil into the scalp and comb through hair.

4. Wrap hair with a shower cap and towel for 3 hours.

5. Rinse thoroughly with lukewarm water, using shampoo if needed.

Overnight Oil Blend for Hair Loss Prevention

This blend uses natural oils to combat hair loss and strengthen hair.

Ingredients

- Equal parts Castor Oil, Rosemary Oil, and/or Almond Oil

Procedure

1. Mix the oils together.

2. Apply to the scalp at night a few times a week for effective results.

3. Optionally, leave the mixture on overnight to enhance scalp healing.

In-Conditioner for Curly Hair

A leave-in conditioner that hydrates and protects curly hair from dryness throughout the day.

Ingredients

- 3 tablespoons Castor Oil

- 1 tablespoon Argan Oil

Procedure

1. Mix the oils and apply to damp hair.

2.   Start from the tips and work your way up, detangling as you go.

3.   Allow to sit for a few minutes before blow-drying.

This blend of argan and castor oils coats each hair strand, trapping moisture and strengthening against damage.

Repairing Hair Mask for Damaged Hair

This hair mask deeply nourishes and repairs damaged hair by utilizing natural proteins and moisture.

Ingredients

- 2 tablespoons Castor Oil

- 1 tablespoon Raw Honey

- 1 Egg Yolk

Procedure

1.   Whip all ingredients together in a clean glass bowl.

2.   Start applying the mixture from the tips of your hair, working your way up to the scalp.

3.   Cover your hair with a shower cap and leave the mask on for 15 to 60 minutes, allowing the proteins and moisture to repair the strands and seal the cuticles.

4.   Wash the mixture out with your favorite shampoo.

Why It's Good for You: Damaged hair benefits from the proteins in egg yolk and castor oil, which strengthen hair cuticles. Honey and castor oil help seal these cuticles, reducing frizziness, split ends, and breakage.

Castor Oil for Beauty and Hair

Castor oil enriches skin and beard hair, stimulating growth and enhancing density for a fuller, shinier appearance.

Procedure

1.   Mix one teaspoon each of Castor oil, Coconut oil, and Shea Butter with two drops of Atlas Cedar essential oil.

2.   Store in an opaque glass container.

3.   Rub a small amount between your hands and massage into the skin and beard hair morning and/or evening, three times a week.

4.   This balm can also be used to nourish hair ends.

Nature Castor Oil Recipes for Body Care

Castor Oil for Eczema Treatment

Eczema On the Scalp, Hand, Feet and Face

Scalp:

Ingredients:

2 tbsp Castor Oil

2 tbsp Coconut Oil

½ tbsp Eucalyptus Oil

3 drops Tea Tree Essential Oil

1 tsp Aloe Vera Gel.

Procedure:

Mix all ingredients and apply to the scalp.

Massage gently, leave for 10 minutes, then rinse with lukewarm water.

Hands:

- Ingredients:

Castor Oil

Amla Powder

Coconut Oil.

- Procedure:

Mix Amla powder with Castor Oil to a smooth consistency.

Massage into the hands for 10-15 minutes to alleviate eczema symptoms.

Feet:

- Ingredients:

Castor Oil

Coconut Oil.

- Procedure: Apply Castor Oil to the feet, cover with cotton socks, and leave for about an hour overnight.

Face:

- Ingredients:

Castor Oil

Avocado Oil

Eucalyptus Oil (1 drop per 5 ml of Castor).

- Procedure: Apply evenly over the face, leave for 10 minutes, then rinse with lukewarm water.

Castor & Sweet Orange Oil for Eczema Scars

Ingredients

- 1 Tablespoon Castor Oil

- 1 Tablespoon Orange Essential Oil

Directions

1. Dilute the oils together.

2. Clean and dry the affected skin before application.

3. Gently massage the oil mixture into the skin and let it air dry naturally.

Coconut & Castor Oil for Eczema Treatment

Ingredients

- 1 Tablespoon Castor Oil

- 1 Tablespoon Virgin Coconut Oil

Directions

1. Blend the oils together.

2. Apply to cleaned skin.

3. Let it dry overnight and rinse the next morning.

Castor Grapeseed Oil Blend to Cure Eczema

Ingredients

- 1 Tablespoon Castor Oil

- 1 Tablespoon Grapeseed Oil

- 2 Drops Tea Tree Essential Oil

- 2 Drops Neem Oil

- 2 Drops Lemongrass Essential Oil

Directions

1. Combine all oils in a bowl.

2. Wash and dry your face.

3. Apply the oil blend to the skin and let it air dry.

Castor Oil for Foot, Hand and Lips Remedies

Spearmint Lip Balm

This hydrating lip balm uses natural ingredients to keep lips moisturized and protected.

Ingredients

- 2 tbsp Castor Oil
- 1 tbsp Cocoa Butter
- 1 tbsp Beeswax Pellets
- 15 drops of Spearmint Essential Oil

Tutorial Steps

1. Melt cocoa butter and beeswax in a double boiler.
2. Add castor oil and stir without overheating.
3. Remove from heat, add spearmint oil, and pour into containers.
4. Allow to solidify for about 30 minutes before use.

Vitamin E Lip Balm

This lip balm provides SPF protection and intense moisture.

Ingredients

- 1 tbsp Castor Oil
- 1 tbsp Coconut Oil
- 1 tbsp Cocoa Butter
- 1 tbsp Beeswax Pellets

- ½ tsp Vitamin E Oil

Chapped Lips Balm

Ingredients

- 5 drops Castor Oil
- 8 drops Almond Oil
- 10 drops Jojoba Oil

Directions

- Combine all oils in a small glass container and apply twice daily.

Dry Lips Balm

Ingredients

- 5 drops Castor Oil
- 8 drops Almond Oil
- 10 drops Mustard Oil

Directions

- Combine all oils in a small glass container and apply during winter months for soft lips.

Fade-Out Pigmentation

This natural oil blend is designed to improve the appearance of skin pigmentation.

Ingredients

- 5 drops Castor Oil
- 8 drops Olive Oil
- 10 drops Jojoba Oil

Directions

1. Mix the oils together and apply directly to the affected area.

2. Gently massage into the skin until fully absorbed.

Cracked Heels Removal

Castor oil's anti-inflammatory and antibacterial properties make it an effective remedy for cracked heels.

Ingredients

- Castor Oil (as needed)

How to Use

1. Warm the castor oil slightly.

2. Apply a thick layer to the affected area and cover with socks.

3. Leave on overnight.

4. Repeat regularly for faster results.

Foot Bath

A soothing foot bath recipe that helps achieve smooth heels.

Ingredients

- Lemon Juice

- Castor Oil

- Geranium Hydrolat

- Jojoba Oil (Hoba)

Directions

1. Mix lemon juice with Black Castor Oil in a 3:1 ratio.

2. Apply the mixture to steamed, slightly damp feet.

3.   Wait for about 30 minutes.

4.   Wash off with warm water and apply geranium hydro late and jojoba oil or another soothing cream.

Note: Proper shoe selection, a balanced diet, and adequate hydration are essential for maintaining smooth heels.

Nature Castor Oil Recipes for Men's Health

Castor Oil for Beard Growth

Eucalyptus and Castor Oil for Beard Growth

Ingredients

*   1 tbsp Castor Oil

*   4 drops Eucalyptus Essential Oil

Procedure

1.   Clean your beard and skin underneath using warm water to open pores.

2.   Dry your beard thoroughly with a towel.

3.   Mix the castor oil and eucalyptus oil in your palm, warm by rubbing hands together.

4.   Apply evenly across your beard from roots to tips and comb through.

5.   Massage using circular motions to increase absorption and stimulate the skin.

6.   Leave the oil on for a few hours or overnight, then wash off.

7.   Repeat regularly to enhance beard growth and health.

Castor Oil with Jojoba Oil for Beard Growth

Ingredients

- 3-5 drops Castor Oil
- 1 tbsp Jojoba Oil

Procedure

1. Clean your beard with warm water and pat dry.
2. Mix the castor and jojoba oils in your palms.
3. Apply to your beard, massaging thoroughly.
4. Place a hot towel over your beard for 5-10 minutes.
5. Remove the oil gently with a towel and finish with a toner.
6. Repeat 1-2 times weekly.

Castor Oil with Almond Oil & Tea Tree Oil for Beard Growth

Ingredients

- 20 Drops Castor Oil
- 1 tbsp Almond Oil
- 3-4 drops Tea Tree Essential Oil

Procedure

1. Clean your beard with warm water and dry it.
2. Blend the oils and apply to your beard.
3. Massage well and leave for an hour.
4. Wash off with a gentle face wash.
5. Use 1-2 times a week for best results.

Castor Oil for Removal of Warts

Simple Castor Oil Application

Ingredients

- Castor Oil

- Cotton ball

Directions

1. Soak a cotton ball in castor oil.

2. Apply it directly to the wart and secure with a bandage.

3. Leave on overnight and repeat nightly until improvement is noticed.

Castor Oil and Baking Soda Paste

Ingredients

- 1 tablespoon Castor Oil

- 1 teaspoon Baking Soda

Directions

1. Mix into a thick paste.

2. Apply to the wart and cover with a bandage overnight.

3. Wash off in the morning and repeat daily until the wart diminishes.

Castor Oil and Garlic Treatment

Ingredients:

1 tablespoon castor oil

1 fresh garlic clove, crushed

Directions:

1. Mix the castor oil with the crushed garlic to form a paste.
2. Apply this paste directly to the wart and cover it with a bandage to keep it in place overnight.
3. In the morning, remove the bandage and cleanse the area thoroughly. Repeat this process nightly until the wart softens and diminishes.

Castor Oil and Apple Cider Vinegar

Ingredients:

Castor oil

Apple cider vinegar

Cotton ball

Directions:

Soak a cotton ball in a blend of castor oil and a few drops of apple cider vinegar.

Secure the soaked cotton ball over the wart using a bandage or tape.

Leave it in place for a few hours or preferably overnight. Perform this treatment daily until the wart begins to peel off.

Castor Oil and Lemon Essential Oil

Ingredients:

1 tablespoon castor oil

2-3 drops lemon essential oil

Directions:

Combine the castor oil with lemon essential oil in a small container.

Apply the oil mixture directly to the wart twice a day.

If necessary, cover the area with a bandage to enhance absorption. Continue this treatment until the wart completely disappears.

Castor Oil Soak

Ingredients:

Warm water

1/4 cup castor oil

Directions:

Fill a small basin with warm water and stir in the castor oil.

Submerge the affected area, such as a foot or hand, in the basin and allow it to soak for 20-30 minutes.

After soaking, gently dry the area and apply a small amount of castor oil directly to the wart. Repeat this soak daily.

Castor Oil for Boosting your Immune

Castor Oil Pack for Lymphatic Health

Ingredients:

Castor oil

Cotton flannel

Plastic wrap

Heating pad or hot water bottle

Directions:

Soak the cotton flannel in castor oil until completely saturated but not dripping.

Place the soaked flannel over the abdomen or other lymphatic areas such as the armpits or groin.

Cover with plastic wrap to prevent oil leakage.

Place a heating pad or hot water bottle over the plastic wrap and leave it on for 45-60 minutes. Repeat 2-3 times a week to aid lymphatic drainage and boost immune function.

Castor Oil and Essential Oil Blend

Ingredients:

2 tablespoons castor oil

3 drops eucalyptus essential oil

3 drops rosemary essential oil

Directions:

Mix castor oil with eucalyptus and rosemary essential oils.

Massage the oil blend onto the chest, neck, and soles of the feet to enhance the immune response.

Apply daily, especially during periods when immune support is needed.

Castor Oil Ginger Warming Massage

Ingredients:

1 tablespoon castor oil

1 teaspoon fresh ginger juice

Directions:

Combine castor oil and fresh ginger juice.

Slightly warm the mixture, then massage into lymph node areas such as the sides of the neck, armpits, and groin.

Use this massage oil daily to stimulate circulation and boost immunity.

Castor Oil Foot Rub

Ingredients:

2 tablespoons castor oil

2 drops thyme essential oil

2 drops lavender essential oil

Directions:

Mix castor oil with thyme and lavender essential oils.

Rub the blend into the soles of the feet at bedtime, cover with socks to enhance absorption.

This treatment is particularly effective before sleep to support overnight immune function.

Castor Oil Abdominal Rub

Ingredients:

2 tablespoons castor oil

2 drops peppermint essential oil

2 drops lemon essential oil

Directions:

Blend castor oil with peppermint and lemon essential oils.

Apply the mixture to the abdomen in gentle circular motions.

Perform this abdominal rub nightly to potentially aid digestion and boost immunity.

Castor Oil Detox Bath

Ingredients:

1/4 cup castor oil

1/4 cup Epsom salts

5 drops ginger essential oil

Directions:

Fill your bathtub with warm water and add the castor oil, Epsom salts, and ginger essential oil.

Soak in the bath for at least 20 minutes to assist body detoxification and enhance lymphatic health.

Conduct this bath 1-2 times a week as a rejuvenating ritual to support overall immune health.

Nature Castor Oil Recipes for Skin Care

Castor Oil for Anti-Aging

Castor & Aloe Vera Gel

Ingredients:

- 1 tbsp of aloe vera gel

- 10 drops of castor oil

- 5 drops of almond oil

Benefits:

Aloe vera is renowned for its anti-aging properties, helping reduce future lines and wrinkles, according to the Baylor College of Medicine. Almond oil improves complexion, skin tone, and hydration, providing a soothing effect.

Instructions:

1.   Combine all ingredients until smooth.

2.   Massage the mixture onto your face using upward strokes for 3-5 minutes.

3.   Leave the mask on your face for 10 minutes.

4.   Remove with warm water or a washcloth.

5.   Follow with your regular skincare routine, including cleanser, toner, serum, and lotion.

Rice Flour, Turmeric Powder & Castor Oil DIY to Firm Up the Skin

Ingredients:

- 1 tbsp of rice flour

- 12 drops of castor oil

- ⅛ tsp of turmeric powder

- Rose water as needed

Benefits:

Rice flour acts as an anti-inflammatory and antioxidant agent, preventing skin aging and reducing UV damage. It promotes skin lightening and improves hair regrowth, while turmeric helps to remove blemishes and wrinkles, according to Healthline.

Instructions:

1.   Combine rice flour, castor oil, and turmeric powder.

2.   Gradually add rose water until it forms a smooth paste.

3.   Apply the mask to your face and neck, leaving it on for 12-15 minutes.

4.   Follow with your regular skincare routine.

Oat Flour, Vegetable Glycerine & Castor Oil DIY to Nourish Mature Skin

Ingredients:

*   1 tbsp oat flour

*   10 drops of castor oil

*   5 drops of vegetable glycerin

*   Warm water as needed

Benefits:

Glycerin is effective in alleviating skin dryness and improving the barrier function of the skin, per a 2017 study. Oat flour helps to soften and moisturize the skin, reducing the appearance of wrinkles, as noted by Healthfully.

Instructions:

1.   Combine oat flour, castor oil, and vegetable glycerin.

2.   Gradually add warm water until a smooth paste forms.

3.   Apply the mask to your face and neck, leaving it on for 12-15 minutes.

4.   Follow with your regular skincare routine.

Avocado, Apple Juice, and Castor Oil Remedy for Firmer Skin

Ingredients:

*   1 tbsp of mashed avocado

*   8 drops of castor oil

*   10 drops of fresh apple juice

Benefits:

Avocado is loaded with antioxidants, such as vitamin C, which help smooth out wrinkles and maintain youthful skin, as noted by WebMD. Apple juice acts as a natural toner and hydrates the skin effectively.

Instructions:

1.   Combine the mashed avocado, castor oil, and apple juice until smooth.

2.   Apply the mixture to your face, massaging it in with upward strokes for 3-5 minutes.

3.   Leave the mixture on your face for 10 minutes.

4.   Remove the mask using warm water or a washcloth.

5.   Continue with your regular skincare routine, including cleanser, toner, serum, and lotion.

Banana, Dark Brown Sugar, and Castor Oil Remedy for Glowing & Ageless Skin

Ingredients:

*   1 tbsp of mashed banana

*   8 drops of castor oil

*   1 tsp of dark brown sugar

Benefits:

Bananas contain silica, which is thought to help increase collagen production, potentially reducing the appearance of wrinkles, according to Healthline. Dark brown sugar acts as a natural exfoliant.

Instructions:

1.   Mix the banana, castor oil, and dark brown sugar until the sugar is dissolved.

2.   Pat the grainy mask onto your skin and gently massage for two minutes using upward strokes.

3.   Rinse the mask off with warm water or a washcloth.

4.   Follow with your skincare routine, including cleanser, toner, serum, and lotion.

Glycerine and Castor Oil for Skin

Ingredients:

- 1 tbsp glycerin

- 1 tbsp castor oil

Directions:

1.   Mix the glycerin and castor oil until well combined.

2.   Apply a small amount to your face, focusing on dry areas.

3.   Massage the serum into your skin in gentle, circular motions.

4.   Allow it to absorb for at least 10 minutes before applying other skincare products.

5.   Use once or twice daily for hydrated and moisturized skin.

Olive Oil and Castor Oil for Skin

Ingredients:

- 1 tbsp castor oil

- 1 tbsp virgin olive oil

Directions:

1.   Blend the olive oil and castor oil in a bowl.

2.   Apply a small amount to your face, especially on dry areas.

3.   Massage the oil into your skin using gentle, circular motions.

4.   Leave on for at least 30 minutes or overnight.

5.   Rinse with warm water and pat dry. Use once or twice a week.

Apple Cider Vinegar and Castor Oil for Skin

Ingredients:

*   1/2 cup water

*   1 tbsp castor oil

*   1 tbsp apple cider vinegar

Directions:

1.   Mix the apple cider vinegar and castor oil.

2.   Add water and stir until evenly distributed.

3.   Transfer to a spray bottle.

4.   Spray on the face after cleansing, avoiding the eyes.

5.   Massage gently into the skin.

6.   Let the toner dry before applying other products.

7.   Use daily for balanced and moisturized skin.

Coconut Oil and Castor Oil for Skin

Ingredients:

*   1 tbsp castor oil

*   1 tbsp virgin coconut oil

Directions:

1.   Mix the coconut oil and castor oil in a bowl.

2.   Apply a small amount to your face, focusing on areas needing extra moisture.

3.   Massage gently in circular motions.

4.   Leave on for at least 30 minutes or overnight.

5.   Rinse with warm water and pat dry. Use once or twice weekly.

Zinc and Castor Oil Cream for Skin Healing

Ingredients:

*   2 tablespoons Castor Oil

*   1 tablespoon Zinc Oxide Powder

Directions:

1.   Mix the zinc oxide powder and castor oil in a small bowl until well combined.

2.   Apply a small amount of the cream to the affected area using gentle, circular motions.

3.   Massage the cream into your skin until it is fully absorbed.

4.   Leave the cream on your skin for at least 30 minutes or overnight, depending on your preference.

5.   Rinse your skin with warm water and pat dry.

6.   Repeat this process once or twice daily to soothe and heal irritated skin.

Sesame and Castor Oil Serum for Skin Nourishment

Ingredients:

*   1 tablespoon Sesame Oil

*   1 tablespoon Castor Oil

Directions:

1.   Mix the sesame oil and castor oil in a small bowl until well combined.

2.   Apply a small amount of the serum to your face using gentle, circular motions.

3.   Massage the serum into your skin until it is fully absorbed.

4.   Leave the serum on your skin for at least 30 minutes or overnight, depending on your preference.

5.   Rinse your face with warm water and pat dry.

Vitamin E and Castor Oil Serum for Antioxidant Protection

Ingredients:

•   1 tablespoon Castor Oil

•   1 tablespoon Vitamin E Oil

Directions:

1.   Mix the vitamin E oil and castor oil in a small bowl until well combined.

2.   Apply a small amount of the serum to your face using gentle, circular motions.

3.   Massage the serum into your skin until it is fully absorbed.

4.   Leave the serum on your skin for at least half an hour or overnight.

5.   Rinse your face with warm water and pat dry.

Avocado and Castor Oil Moisturizer for Enhanced Hydration

Ingredients:

•   1 tablespoon Castor Oil

•   1 tablespoon Avocado Oil

Directions:

1.   Mix the avocado oil and castor oil in a small bowl until well combined.

2.   Apply a small amount of moisturizer to your face, using gentle, circular motions.

3.   Massage the moisturizer into your skin until it is fully absorbed.

4.   Leave the moisturizer on your skin for at least 30 minutes or overnight, depending on your preference.

5.   Rinse your face with warm water and pat dry. Repeat this process once or twice weekly to keep your skin moisturized and healthy.

Castor Oil Treatments for Acne

Castor Oil Steam Cleanse

What You Will Need:

- A soup pot filled with water

- 1 or 2 teaspoons Castor oil

- A towel

- Mild exfoliating cleansing cream

Method:

1.   Boil water in a pot and then remove from heat.

2.   Drape a towel over your head and steam your face comfortably for up to 5 minutes.

3.   Soak a towel in warm water, wring it out, and massage your face to clean out your pores.

4.   Add castor oil onto the soaked cloth and massage over your face again in gentle circular motions.

5.   Wash your face with cold water and pat dry.

6.   Apply two drops of castor oil on your face and leave it overnight.

7.   Clean it off in the morning with a mild exfoliating cleansing cream.

Why This Works:

The steam opens your pores, allowing the castor oil to penetrate deeply and moisturize, exfoliate, and nourish your skin, which helps prevent and treat acne.

Plain Castor Oil Application

What You Will Need:

- Castor Oil

Method:

1. Test castor oil on a small area of your skin to ensure there is no irritation.

2. Wash your face with a gentle cleanser and pat it dry.

3. Massage castor oil onto the affected areas of your skin for 5-10 minutes.

4. Leave it on for an hour before washing off your face.

5. Repeat this procedure twice a day for effective results.

Castor Oil and Olive Oil

What You Will Need:

- 1 teaspoon Olive Oil
- 2 teaspoons Castor Oil

Method:

1. Mix olive oil and castor oil in a bowl.

2. Apply and gently massage it on your face.

3. Leave it on for about half an hour or overnight.

4. In the morning, use an exfoliating scrub to remove it and pat dry.

Why This Works:

Olive oil mixed with castor oil deeply cleanses and hydrates the skin, removing dirt and impurities from pores and reducing acne outbreaks.

Castor Oil, Almond Oil, and Camphor Oil Treatment for Skin

Ingredients:

*   1/2 cup Castor Oil

*   1/2 cup Almond Oil (recommend Avaya's Almond Oil for its high antioxidant content)

*   1 teaspoon Camphor Oil

Preparation Time: Approximately 5 minutes to measure and mix the oils.

Treatment Time: Overnight for best results.

Method:

1.   Mix the castor oil, almond oil, and camphor oil together in a mixing bowl.

2.   Wash and dry your face thoroughly before applying the oil blend.

3.   Apply the oil mixture using your fingertips, massaging gently into your skin.

4.   Leave the treatment on your face overnight.

5.   Wash off in the morning with a mild exfoliating cleansing cream.

Frequency: Apply nightly before bed for as long as needed to clear up acne.

Why It Works: Almond oil nourishes the skin due to its rich content of antioxidants and omega-3 fatty acids. Castor oil acts as an effective antioxidant, rejuvenating the skin, while camphor oil provides a cooling effect and helps reduce skin irritation.

Castor Oil and Zinc Treatment for Acne

Ingredients:

- 8 tablespoons Castor Oil

- 2 tablespoons Beeswax

- 1 tablespoon Zinc Oxide

- Essential oil (optional - such as Lavender or Coconut oil)

Preparation Time: About 15 minutes.

Treatment Time: Overnight application.

Method:

1. Melt the beeswax into the castor oil using a double boiler.

2. Mix in the zinc oxide once the wax has melted.

3. Add an essential oil of your choice for additional benefits and fragrance.

4. Store the mixture in a jar.

5. Apply to the acne-affected spots on your face and leave it overnight.

6. Wash off with cold water in the morning.

Frequency: Use nightly before bed.

Why It Works: Zinc is effective in fighting bacteria and reducing inflammation. It also helps fade acne scars, while castor oil moisturizes and heals the skin.

Castor Oil and Grapeseed Oil Treatment for Acne

Ingredients:

- Equal parts Castor Oil and Grapeseed Oil

- 2 drops of Tea Tree, Lemongrass, or Neem Oil

- Apple Cider Vinegar

- Cotton Balls

Preparation Time: 15 minutes.

Treatment Time: Overnight.

Method:

1. Mix castor oil and grapeseed oil in equal quantities.

2. Add two drops of either tea tree, lemongrass, or neem oil and stir well.

3. Apply the mixture to your face like a mask and massage gently for about 5 minutes.

4. Leave it overnight.

5. In the morning, heat a washcloth in hot water, squeeze out the excess, and place it on your face for about 10 minutes in intervals.

6. Wipe off the excess oil using apple cider vinegar on a cotton ball.

Frequency: Daily use.

Why It Works: Grapeseed oil is light and easily absorbed, making it excellent for skin prone to acne. Combined with the antibacterial properties of tea tree, lemongrass, or neem oil, and the deep cleansing action of castor oil, this treatment effectively fights acne.

Castor Oil and Baking Soda Mask for Acne

Ingredients:

- 1 tablespoon Castor Oil
- 1 tablespoon Baking Soda

Preparation Time: 5 minutes.

Treatment Time: 15-20 minutes.

Method:

1. Clean your face and pat it dry.

2. Mix castor oil and baking soda to form a paste.

3.	Apply the mixture to the acne-affected areas on your face and neck.

4.	Leave it on for about 15-20 minutes before rinsing it off with a gentle exfoliating cream and cold water.

Frequency: Daily.

Why It Works: Baking soda has anti-inflammatory and antiseptic properties that help dry out acne and cool down inflamed skin, while castor oil provides hydration and nourishment.

Castor Oil and Jojoba Oil Treatment

Ingredients:

•	1 teaspoon Castor Oil

•	3 teaspoons Jojoba Oil (consider Avaya's Jojoba Oil for high quality)

Preparation Time: 5 minutes.

Treatment Time: 5 minutes.

Method:

1.	Mix castor oil with jojoba oil in a bowl.

2.	Splash water on your face, pat it dry, then apply the oil mixture.

3.	Place a hot washcloth over your face for a minute or two to enhance absorption.

4.	Rinse your face with cold water and pat dry.

Frequency: Regular use.

Why It Works: Jojoba oil mimics the skin's natural oils and helps regulate sebum production, while castor oil provides deep moisture and healing properties.

Castor Oil and Turmeric Treatment for Acne

Ingredients:

- 1/2 teaspoon Castor Oil

- 1 teaspoon Turmeric Powder

Preparation Time: 2-3 minutes.

Treatment Time: 15-20 minutes.

Method:

1. Wash your face and pat it dry.

2. Mix castor oil with turmeric powder in a bowl.

3. Apply the mixture to the affected areas on your face and neck.

4. Leave it on for about 15-20 minutes.

5. Rinse off with cold water and pat your skin dry.

Frequency: Once daily.

Why It Works: Turmeric is a powerful antibacterial and anti-inflammatory agent that fights acne-causing bacteria and helps reduce inflammation. It also helps to fade old acne scars.

Castor Oil and Organic Coconut Oil for Acne

Ingredients:

- 3 teaspoons Castor Oil

- 8 teaspoons Organic Coconut Oil

Preparation Time: 5 minutes.

Treatment Time: Can be left on for 20 minutes or overnight.

Method:

1.   Boil water, then remove from heat.

2.   Drape a towel over your head and steam your face over the pot for 5-10 minutes to open pores.

3.   Mix castor oil and coconut oil in another bowl.

4.   Apply this oil mixture gently to your face.

5.   Leave the mask on overnight.

6.   Remove with a wet cloth in the morning.

7.   Cleanse your face with a mild exfoliating cream and pat dry.

Frequency: Daily for one month, or until the acne clears up.

Why It Works: Coconut oil contains lauric acid, which has antibacterial properties that help fight acne-causing bacteria. Castor oil enhances moisture content in the skin, reducing the appearance of scars and aiding in the repair of damaged skin.

Castor Oil for Acne Scars

Ingredients:

*   2 tablespoons Jamaican Black Castor Oil

*   2 tablespoons Grapeseed Oil

Instructions:

1.   Mix both oils in a bowl.

2.   Apply the mixture to the skin where acne scars are present.

3.   Gently massage the oils into the skin to moisturize and help lighten acne scars, as grapeseed oil has properties that can fight acne.

4.   Leave on as an overnight treatment for best results.

Dead Skin Remover

Ingredients:

- 3 tablespoons Pure Castor Oil

- 2 tablespoons Almond Oil

Instructions:

1. Combine castor oil and almond oil in a bowl.

2. Apply the oil mixture to areas with dead skin.

3. Massage gently to cleanse the skin and remove dead skin layers.

4. Leave on for a few hours or overnight for deep nourishment and smoothing of the skin.

Castor Oil Facial and Body Moisturizer

Essential Oil Facial Scrub

Ingredients:

- 1 tablespoon Organic Castor Oil

- 1 tablespoon Organic Coconut Oil

- 1/4 teaspoon to 2 teaspoons Baking Soda (adjust based on skin sensitivity)

- 1 to 5 drops each of Lemon Oil, Lavender Oil, Cedarwood Oil, and Frankincense Oil

Instructions:

1. Combine all ingredients in a small bowl and mix until well combined.

2. Transfer the scrub to a small glass jar and let it sit for a couple of days.

3. To use: Apply on dry or very slightly damp skin. Gently scrub all over the face, avoiding the eye area.

4. Wet a washcloth with warm water, wring it out, and lay over your face to steam and remove impurities.

5.   Rinse thoroughly using the cloth 3-4 times until all traces of the cleanser are removed.

6.   Pat face dry with a towel.

Castor & Aloe Vera Gel for Anti-Aging

Ingredients:

- 1 tablespoon Aloe Vera Gel

- 10 drops Castor Oil

- 5 drops Almond Oil

Instructions:

1.   Mix all ingredients until smooth.

2.   Massage onto your face using upward strokes for 3-5 minutes.

3.   Leave the mask on your face for 10 minutes.

4.   Remove with warm water or a washcloth.

5.   Follow up with your regular skincare routine.

Castor Oil Cuticle Cream

Ingredients:

- 1 tablespoon Castor Oil

- 1/2 tablespoon Honey

- 1 tablespoon Beeswax

Instructions:

1.   Combine all ingredients in a pan and heat on low until melted and well mixed.

2.   Pour the mixture into a glass jar and let it cool and solidify.

3.   Apply nightly to nails and surrounding skin to moisturize and strengthen nails, as well as prevent fungal infections.

Chocolate Orange Lip Balm

Ingredients:

- 10g Natural Yellow Beeswax

- 10.5g Organic Cocoa Butter

- 14g Castor Oil

- 15g Macadamia Nut Oil

- 0.25g High Strength Vitamin E

- 0.25g Orange Essential Oil (approximately 4 drops)

Instructions:

1.   Melt beeswax and cocoa butter in a heatproof bowl, either in the microwave or using a double boiler.

2.   Remove from heat and stir in macadamia nut oil, castor oil, vitamin E, and orange essential oil.

3.   Pour into lip balm containers.

4.   Allow to set, optionally in the fridge for faster setting.

5.   Use as needed for hydrated and glossy lips.

Castor Oil Night-time Facial Serum

Ingredients:

- 1 tablespoon Argan Oil

- 1 tablespoon Castor Oil

- 1 teaspoon Rosehip Seed Oil

- A few drops of Geranium Essential Oil

Instructions:

1. Mix argan oil, castor oil, and rosehip seed oil in a small container.
2. Add a few drops of geranium essential oil for fragrance.
3. Shake well to combine.
4. Apply to clean, toned skin before bedtime, massaging gently.
5. Note: Best for nighttime use due to its rich consistency.

Castor Oil Face Cleanser

Ingredients:

- 2 tablespoons Castor Oil
- 1 tablespoon Carrier Oil (Jojoba, Olive, or Coconut)
- 5-10 drops of Essential Oil (Lavender, Tea Tree, or Chamomile)

Instructions:

1. Mix the castor and carrier oils.
2. Add essential oils for additional benefits and fragrance.
3. Massage onto your face in circular motions.
4. Use a warm, wet washcloth to steam and remove the oil.

Oil Cleanser for Oily and Acne-Prone Skin

Ingredients:

- ½ teaspoon Castor Oil
- ½ teaspoon Jojoba Oil

Instructions:

1. Blend the oils in a glass bowl.
2. Massage the oil blend on your face for 3-5 minutes.

3.	Place a warm microfiber towel on your face to help dissolve impurities.

4.	Wipe off with the same towel, then cleanse gently with apple cider vinegar.

Castor Oil Moisturizer Recipe

Ingredients:

*	2/3 cup Castor Oil

*	1/3 cup Grapefruit Seed Extract

*	5-10 drops of an Essential Oil blend

Instructions:

1.	Combine castor oil and grapefruit seed extract in a container.

2.	Add essential oils and mix thoroughly.

3.	Apply to clean skin. Can be used on the face or body.

Castor Oil Moisturizing Mask

Ingredients:

*	1 tablespoon Castor Oil

*	1 tablespoon Honey

*	1 Egg Yolk (optional)

Instructions:

1.	Combine castor oil, honey, and egg yolk (if using).

2.	Apply to a clean face and avoid the eye area.

3.	Leave on for 15-20 minutes.

4.   Rinse with lukewarm water and follow with moisturizer.

Rice Flour, Turmeric Powder & Castor Oil Mask for Firming Skin

Ingredients:

- 1 tbsp Rice Flour
- 12 drops Castor Oil
- ⅛ tsp Turmeric Powder
- Rose Water (as needed)

Benefits: Rice flour and turmeric have anti-inflammatory and antioxidant properties that help prevent skin aging and improve skin tone. Castor oil helps in skin regeneration.

Instructions:

1.   Mix rice flour, castor oil, and turmeric powder.
2.   Gradually add rose water until a smooth paste forms.
3.   Apply to your face and neck for 12-15 minutes.
4.   Rinse off and follow up with your skincare routine.

Oat Flour, Vegetable Glycerine & Castor Oil Mask for Mature Skin

Ingredients:

- 1 tbsp Oat Flour
- 10 drops Castor Oil
- 5 drops Vegetable Glycerin
- Warm Water (as needed)

Benefits: Oat flour softens and moisturizes the skin, reducing wrinkles. Glycerin improves skin's barrier function and alleviates dryness.

Instructions:

1. Combine oat flour, castor oil, and vegetable glycerin.

2. Slowly add warm water to achieve a smooth consistency.

3. Apply the mask to your face and neck for 12-15 minutes.

4. Rinse off and proceed with your usual skincare routine.

Avocado, Apple Juice, and Castor Oil Mask for Firmer Skin

Ingredients:

- 1 tbsp mashed Avocado

- 8 drops Castor Oil

- 10 drops Fresh Apple Juice

Benefits: Avocado contains antioxidants like vitamin C to reduce wrinkles. Apple juice acts as a natural toner and hydrates the skin.

Instructions:

1. Mix all ingredients until smooth.

2. Massage onto your face for 3-5 minutes using upward strokes.

3. Leave on for 10 minutes, then rinse with warm water.

4. Follow with your regular skincare routine.

Banana, Dark Brown Sugar & Castor Oil Mask for Glowing Skin

Ingredients:

- 1 tbsp mashed Banana

- 8 drops Castor Oil

- 1 tsp Dark Brown Sugar

Benefits: Bananas can increase collagen due to their silica content, potentially reducing wrinkles. Dark brown sugar acts as a natural exfoliant.

Instructions:

1. Combine all ingredients until the sugar dissolves.

2. Pat onto your skin and gently massage for two minutes.

3. Rinse off with warm water and continue with your skincare routine.

Olive Oil and Castor Oil Facial Oil

Ingredients:

- 1 tbsp Castor Oil

- 1 tbsp Virgin Olive Oil

Benefits: Both oils are rich in antioxidants and fatty acids, nourishing and moisturizing the skin.

Instructions:

1. Mix the oils together.

2. Apply to the face, especially on dry areas, and massage in circular motions.

3. Leave on for at least 30 minutes or overnight.

4. Rinse off with warm water and pat dry.

Apple Cider Vinegar and Castor Oil Toner

Ingredients:

- ½ Cup Water

- 1 tbsp Castor Oil

- 1 tbsp Apple Cider Vinegar

Benefits: Apple cider vinegar helps unclog pores and exfoliate, while castor oil moisturizes and nourishes the skin.

Instructions:

1.   Mix all ingredients and transfer to a spray bottle.

2.   Spray onto cleansed face, avoiding the eyes.

3.   Allow the toner to dry before proceeding with your skincare routine.

Coconut Oil and Castor Oil Facial Oil

Ingredients:

*   1 tablespoon Castor Oil

*   1 tablespoon Virgin Coconut Oil

Directions:

1.   Mix the coconut oil and castor oil in a small bowl until well combined.

2.   Apply a small amount to your face, focusing on dry areas or those needing extra moisture.

3.   Massage the oil into your skin using gentle, circular motions.

4.   Leave the oil on your skin for at least 30 minutes or overnight for deeper moisturization.

5.   Rinse your face with warm water and pat dry.

6.   Repeat once or twice weekly to keep your skin moisturized and protected.

Zinc and Castor Oil Skin Cream

Ingredients:

*   2 tablespoons Castor Oil

*   1 tablespoon Zinc Oxide Powder

Directions:

1.   Mix the zinc oxide powder and castor oil in a small bowl until well combined.

2.   Apply a small amount of the cream to the affected area, using gentle, circular motions.

3.   Massage the cream into your skin until fully absorbed.

4.   Leave on for at least 30 minutes or overnight, depending on your preference.

5.   Rinse with warm water and pat dry.

6.   Use once or twice daily to soothe and heal irritated skin.

Sesame Oil and Castor Oil Skin Serum

Ingredients:

- 1 tablespoon Sesame Oil
- 1 tablespoon Castor Oil

Directions:

1.   Mix the sesame oil and castor oil in a small bowl until well combined.

2.   Apply a small amount of the serum to your face using gentle, circular motions.

3.   Massage the serum into your skin until it is fully absorbed.

4.   Leave the serum on your skin for at least 30 minutes or overnight.

5.   Rinse your face with warm water and pat dry.

Vitamin E and Castor Oil Skin Serum

Ingredients:

- 1 tablespoon Castor Oil
- 1 tablespoon Vitamin E Oil

Directions:

1. Mix the vitamin E oil and castor oil in a small bowl until well combined.

2. Apply a small amount of the serum to your face using gentle, circular motions.

3. Massage the serum into your skin until it is fully absorbed.

4. Leave on for at least half an hour or overnight.

5. Rinse your face with warm water and pat dry.

Avocado Oil and Castor Oil Moisturizer

Ingredients:

*   1 tablespoon Castor Oil

*   1 tablespoon Avocado Oil

Directions:

1. Mix the avocado oil and castor oil in a small bowl until well combined.

2. Apply a small amount of moisturizer to your face, using gentle, circular motions.

3. Massage the moisturizer into your skin until it is fully absorbed.

4. Leave on for at least 30 minutes or overnight.

5. Rinse your face with warm water and pat dry.

6. Repeat once or twice weekly.

Castor Oil and Lemon Juice for Skin Whitening

Ingredients:

*   1 teaspoon Castor Oil

*   2 teaspoons Honey

- ½ teaspoon Lemon Juice

Directions:

1. Mix castor oil, honey, and freshly squeezed lemon juice in a bowl.

2. Apply to a cleansed face.

3. Leave on for 15-20 minutes before rinsing with water.

Castor Oil and Tea Tree Essential Oil for Skin Health

Ingredients:

- ½ teaspoon Castor Oil

- 1 teaspoon Golden Jojoba Oil

- 2 drops Tea Tree Essential Oil

Directions:

1. Mix castor oil, jojoba oil, and tea tree oil.

2. Apply gently to cleansed skin.

3. Leave on for several minutes.

4. Remove immediately if you experience any irritation.

Castor Oil for Mole Removal

Castor oil is an effective natural remedy for removing moles. It's combined with other ingredients to enhance its efficacy. Here are several methods to use castor oil for mole removal, each with specific ingredients and procedures.

Castor Oil and Garlic

Ingredients:

- Three drops of castor oil

- Half a teaspoon of garlic powder or a teaspoon of fresh garlic paste

- A mixing bowl

- A towel

Directions:

- Combine the castor oil with garlic powder or paste in a bowl to form a thick paste.

- Apply the paste to the mole and leave it on for a few hours.

- Rinse off with water and pat the area dry with a towel.

Process Time:

- For best results, apply this paste twice daily for at least a week.

Castor Oil and Honey

Ingredients:

- A teaspoon of honey

- Three drops of castor oil

- An adhesive bandage

- Soap

- A towel

- A bowl for mixing

Directions:

- Clean the mole area with soap and dry thoroughly.

- Mix the honey and castor oil in a bowl.

- Apply the mixture to the mole and cover with a bandage for up to three hours.

- Remove the bandage, clean the area, and reapply the mixture.

- Rinse off after another three hours.

Process Time:

- Use this method twice daily for a week for noticeable results.

Castor Oil and Tea Tree Oil

Ingredients:

- Three drops of tea tree oil

- One teaspoon of castor oil

- Cotton

- Adhesive tape

- A bowl for mixing

Directions:

- Mix the oils in a bowl.

- Soak the cotton in the oil mixture and place it on the mole.

- Secure it with adhesive tape and leave for 3 to 4 hours.

Process Time:

- Results can appear from one week to one month, depending on the mole's size. Apply twice daily.

Castor Oil and Baking Soda

Ingredients:

- Three drops of castor oil

- Baking soda

- Adhesive bandages

- A mixing bowl

Directions:

- In a bowl, mix castor oil with enough baking soda to form a sticky paste.

- Apply to the mole and cover with adhesive bandages to keep the paste in place.

- Remove the bandage and wash off after 8 hours.

Process Time:

- Apply every other evening, preferably overnight, and results can be seen in two to three weeks.

Castor Oil and Grape Seed Extract

Ingredients:

- 3-4 drops of grape seed extract

- 1 teaspoon of castor oil

- A mixing bowl

Directions:

- Combine the extract and oil in a bowl.

- Generously apply the mixture to the mole and leave it on for several hours, up to eight.

- Rinse off with water later.

Process Time:

- Results should be visible in two to three weeks if used two to three times daily.

Castor Oil and Apple Cider Vinegar

Ingredients:

- 1 teaspoon of apple cider vinegar
- 1 teaspoon of castor oil
- A bowl for mixing
- A cotton pad

Directions:

- Mix the apple cider vinegar and castor oil in a bowl.
- Soak a cotton pad in the mixture and gently wipe the mole.

Process Time:

- Repeat twice daily for a week for effective results.

Castor Oil and Flaxseed Oil

Ingredients:

- 1 teaspoon of castor oil
- 1 teaspoon of flaxseed oil
- A bowl for mixing
- A cotton balls

Directions:

- Mix the oils in a bowl.
- Soak a cotton ball in the mixture and apply it to the mole.

Process Time:

- Flaxseed accelerates healing, and moles may fall off within days of twice-daily applications.

Castor Oil and Frankincense Oil

Ingredients:

- A few drops of frankincense oil

- 1 teaspoon of castor oil

- A cotton balls

- A bowl for mixing

Directions:

- Combine the oils in a bowl.

- Soak a cotton ball in the mixture and apply it to the mole for up to four hours.

Process Time:

- Frankincense's astringent properties may take two to three weeks to remove moles if used twice or thrice daily.

Castor Oil for Reducing Dark Spots

Dark spots can detract from your skin's natural beauty. Using castor oil is an effective way to lighten these spots and give your skin a fresher look. This natural remedy is gentle on the skin and free from harmful side effects.

Castor Oil and Turmeric Powder

Ingredients:

- 1 teaspoon castor oil

- 1/2 teaspoon turmeric powder

Directions:

- Combine the castor oil and turmeric powder in a small bowl. Adjust the turmeric quantity to achieve a thicker consistency if desired.

- Apply the mixture to the dark spots and leave it on for one hour.

- Rinse your face with lukewarm water.

- Use daily until you see the desired improvements.

Turmeric is renowned for its skin health benefits, particularly in treating dark spots and hyperpigmentation.

Castor Oil and Vitamin E

Ingredients:

- 1 teaspoon castor oil

- 1 Vitamin E capsule

Directions:

- Extract the oil from the Vitamin E capsule and mix it with the castor oil.

- Apply the blend all over your face.

- Massage gently in upward circular motions, concentrating on dark spots, for 5 to 10 minutes.

- Wash off with a facial cleanser.

- Apply twice daily for best results.

Vitamin E helps to even out skin tone, and its combination with castor oil is particularly effective in fading dark spots quickly.

Castor Oil and Lemon Juice

Ingredients:

- 1 teaspoon castor oil

- 1/2 teaspoon lemon juice

- 1 teaspoon honey

Directions:

- Mix all ingredients in a bowl.
- Apply the mixture to the affected areas or use as a full facial mask for 30 minutes.
- Wash off with lukewarm water and a gentle cleanser.
- Apply once daily.

Castor Oil and Zinc Oxide

Ingredients:

- 1 teaspoon castor oil
- 15 grams zinc oxide powder

Directions:

- Combine the castor oil and zinc oxide powder until a paste forms.
- Apply to dark spots and leave for one hour.
- Rinse with lukewarm water.
- Use three times a week.

Castor Oil and Grapeseed Oil

Ingredients:

- 1 teaspoon castor oil
- 1 tablespoon grapeseed oil

Directions:

- Blend the oils together thoroughly.
- Massage into your face in a circular motion for 3 minutes.
- Place a warm, damp towel over your face to enhance absorption.
- Once the towel cools, use it to wipe off the excess oil.

Castor Oil and Sunflower Oil

Ingredients:

- 1 teaspoon castor oil
- 3 teaspoons sunflower oil

Directions:

- Mix the oils well.
- Massage onto your face and leave for 10 minutes.
- Rinse with lukewarm water or cleanse with a warm towel.

DIY Castor Oil Remedy

Ingredients:

- 1 tablespoon fuller's earth
- 1 teaspoon castor oil
- 1 teaspoon fresh lemon juice

Directions:

- Mix to form a smooth paste, adding water if necessary.
- Apply to the entire face or directly on dark spots.
- Leave for 15-20 minutes and rinse off.

Castor Oil for Stretch Mark Removal

Castor Oil and Cloves

Castor Oil and Cloves Clove oil is known for its anti-inflammatory and antioxidant properties, which may help remodel skin tissue and reduce scars, although scientific evidence is limited.

You Will Need:

- 2-3 drops of clove essential oil
- 1 tablespoon of cold-pressed castor oil

Method:

1. Combine the oils.
2. Massage into stretch marks.
3. Leave overnight.
4. Apply daily.

Castor Oil and Plastic Wrap

This method may deeply moisturize and reduce the appearance of stretch marks.

You Will Need:

- 1 tablespoon of cold-pressed castor oil
- Cling wrap

Method:

1. Warm the castor oil slightly.
2. Apply to stretch marks.
3. Tightly wrap the area with cling wrap.

4.   Leave for at least 30 minutes.

5.   Unwrap and massage the area again.

6.   Leave the oil on to absorb into the skin.

7.   Repeat daily.

Castor Oil and Sugar Scrub for Stretch Marks

Sugar's coarse texture makes it an ideal natural scrub. While no definitive proof exists that scrubbing reduces stretch marks, many people use sugar scrubs to lessen the appearance of scars.

You Will Need:

*   2 tablespoons of granulated sugar

*   1 tablespoon of cold-pressed castor oil

Method:

1.   Combine the sugar and castor oil to make a scrub.

2.   Massage the scrub onto the stretch marks for 5-10 minutes.

3.   Let it sit for another 15-20 minutes.

4.   Rinse off and apply moisturizer.

5.   Repeat every other day for gradual improvement.

Castor Oil and Oatmeal Pack

Research has shown that colloidal oat extracts can improve skin dryness and texture.

You Will Need:

*   2 tablespoons of ground oatmeal

*   1/2 cup water (50 mL)

- 1 tablespoon of cold-pressed castor oil

Method:

1. Mix the ground oatmeal with water to achieve a paste-like consistency.

2. Stir in the castor oil.

3. Massage the mixture onto stretch marks for 10-15 minutes.

4. Allow it to dry for at least half an hour.

5. Wash off and apply moisturizer.

6. Repeat daily for best results.

Castor Oil and Potato Juice

Although scientific evidence is lacking, anecdotal reports suggest potato juice may reduce the visibility of stretch marks.

You Will Need:

- 1 tablespoon of raw potato juice

- 1 tablespoon of cold-pressed castor oil

Method:

1. Mix the castor oil and potato juice.

2. Massage the mixture onto the stretch marks.

3. Leave it on for half an hour.

4. Wash off and apply moisturizer.

5. Repeat daily.

Turmeric & Castor Oil

The anti-inflammatory and antioxidant properties of turmeric, when combined with castor oil, help reduce stretch marks.

Ingredients:

- ½ tsp Turmeric
- 1 tsp Castor Oil

Method:

1. Mix turmeric and castor oil in a bowl.
2. Massage the mixture onto stretch marks.
3. Leave for an hour then rinse off. Follow with moisturizer.
4. Note: Turmeric may stain skin and clothes.

Aloe Vera Gel & Castor Oil

Aloe Vera gel boosts collagen production and moisturizes, enhancing the skin-conditioning effects of castor oil.

Ingredients:

- 1 tsp Aloe Vera Gel
- 1 tsp Castor Oil

Method:

1. Combine aloe vera gel and castor oil in a bowl.
2. Apply to stretch marks and leave until absorbed.
3. Can be applied daily for faster results.

Almond Oil & Castor Oil

Combining almond oils with castor oil creates an effective remedy for reducing and preventing stretch marks.

Ingredients:

- 1 tbsp Castor Oil

- 1 tbsp Sweet Almond Oil

- 3-4 drops Bitter Almond Essential Oil

Method:

1. Mix all ingredients in a bowl.

2. Massage onto stretch marks.

3. Leave for an hour or overnight. Repeat daily.

Castor Oil for Skin Pigmentation

Castor Oil and Turmeric

This combination works effectively against skin pigmentation while evening out skin tone.

Ingredients:

- 3-4 drops of castor oil

- 1 tablespoon of turmeric powder

Procedure:

1. Mix castor oil with turmeric powder in a bowl.

2. Apply the paste to your face, massaging gently.

3. Leave the mask on for 15-20 minutes.

4. Rinse with lukewarm water.

Castor Oil and Vitamin E Oil

Vitamin E reduces skin inflammation and, along with castor oil, clears blemishes.

Ingredients:

- 1 tbsp of castor oil
- 4 drops of Vitamin E oil

Procedure:

1. Combine the oils in a bowl.

2. Apply the mixture to your face, massaging gently in circular and upward motions.

3. Leave for 10-15 minutes, then rinse with lukewarm water.

Fullers Earth and Castor Oil for Enhanced Skin Texture

Fullers Earth, also known as Multani Mitti, is renowned for improving skin texture and brightening the complexion. It helps enhance skin tone and combats marks and blemishes while absorbing excess oil for clearer skin.

Ingredients:

- 10 grams of Multani Mitti (Fullers Earth)
- 10 ml Castor Oil
- 4 drops of Vitamin E oil

Procedure:

1. In a bowl, mix Multani Mitti and castor oil to form a smooth paste. Add a few drops of Vitamin E oil.

2. Apply the mask evenly across your face, starting from the forehead to the cheeks and down to the neck.

3. Allow the mask to dry for 30-40 minutes.

4.   Rinse off with lukewarm water, pat dry, and follow up with a moisturizing cream to counteract the drying effects of Multani Mitti.

Natural Castor Oil Recipes for Pet Skin and Coat Health

Castor oil can be beneficial for pets' skin and coat health but should be used with caution. Always consult a veterinarian before introducing new treatments.

Castor Oil Coat Enhancer

Ingredients:

*   1 tablespoon castor oil

*   1 tablespoon coconut oil

Directions:

1.   Combine the oils until well blended.

2.   Apply a small amount to your pet's coat to enhance shine and moisturize the skin.

3.   Use sparingly to avoid a greasy coat. Apply weekly or as needed.

Castor Oil Paw Pad Softener

Ingredients:

*   Castor oil

Directions:

1.   Apply a small amount of castor oil to a clean cloth.

2.   Gently rub the oil into your pet's paw pads at bedtime to allow absorption overnight.

Castor Oil and Lavender Itch Relief

Ingredients:

*   2 tablespoons castor oil

*   1 drop lavender essential oil (therapeutic grade and pet-safe)

Directions:

1.   Mix the oils and apply to dry or itchy areas of your pet's skin.

2.   Use sparingly and watch for any adverse reactions.

Castor Oil Wound Care

Ingredients:

*   Castor oil

*   Clean cotton ball

Directions:

1.   Clean the minor cut or scrape with vet-approved methods.

2.   Apply a small amount of castor oil with a cotton ball.

3.   Use only on minor wounds and consult a vet for serious injuries.

Castor Oil Ear Mite Treatment

Ingredients:

*   2 tablespoons castor oil

- 1 tablespoon olive oil

Directions:

1.   Mix the oils and use a dropper to apply a few drops into the ear canal.

2.   Massage gently and repeat daily for a week under veterinary guidance.

Castor Oil Flea Repellent

Ingredients:

- 2 tablespoons castor oil

- 2 tablespoons water

- 2 drops peppermint essential oil (pet-safe)

Directions:

1.   Combine ingredients in a spray bottle.

2.   Spray lightly on your pet's coat before going outdoors, avoiding sensitive areas.

Natural Castor Oil Recipes for Pain and Inflammation Relief

Castor Oil for Muscle and Joint Pain

Castor Oil for Arthritis Pain Relief

Ingredients

- Castor oil

- Cotton pads

Directions:

1.   Warm the castor oil to a lukewarm temperature.

2.   Massage the oil into the affected area thoroughly.

3.   Apply a hot pack afterward.

4.   Use this treatment on alternate days for pain relief.

Castor Oil for Knee Pain

Ingredients:

- Castor oil
- Hot water pack
- Cotton pads

Directions:

1.   Soak cotton pads in lukewarm castor oil overnight.

2.   Squeeze excess oil from the pads.

3.   Massage over the painful area and apply a hot water pack.

4.   Repeat daily.

Castor Oil and Flannel for Painful Joints

Ingredients:

- Flannel cloth
- 20 ml Castor oil
- Plastic wrap
- Towel

- Hot water pack

Directions:

1.   Warm 20 ml of castor oil and soak the folded flannel in it for 20 minutes.

2.   Place the flannel over the affected joint and wrap with plastic to secure.

3.   Leave the castor oil pack on for 30-45 minutes for deep relief.

Castor Oil Backache Remedy

Ingredients:

- Castor oil (as needed)

- A clean and soft cloth

- Hot water bag

How to Use:

1.   Apply castor oil topically over the back.

2.   Place the cloth over the oiled area and then the hot water bag on top.

3.   If the bag is too hot, wrap it in a towel to protect your skin.

4.   Leave in place for an hour to allow the oil to penetrate deeply.

5.   Massage the area to further relieve pain.

Castor Oil Muscle Relief Massage Blend

Ingredients:

- 3 tablespoons castor oil

- 5 drops eucalyptus essential oil

- 5 drops rosemary essential oil

Directions:

1. Mix the castor oil with eucalyptus and rosemary essential oils.

2. Massage this blend into sore muscles to reduce tension and discomfort.

Castor Oil and Turmeric Anti-Inflammatory Wrap

Ingredients:

- 2 tablespoons castor oil

- 1 teaspoon turmeric powder

- 1/2 teaspoon black pepper

Directions:

1. Combine castor oil, turmeric, and black pepper to create a paste.

2. Apply to the affected area and wrap with a cloth.

3. Leave on for 1-2 hours or overnight to help reduce inflammation.

Castor Oil Hot Compress for Muscle Pain

Ingredients:

- Castor oil

- A clean cloth

- Hot water bottle or heating pad

Directions:

1. Soak the cloth in castor oil and place over the sore area.

2. Cover with plastic wrap, then place a hot water bottle or heating pad on top for 30-60 minutes.

Soothing Castor Oil Bath

Ingredients:

- 1/4 cup castor oil
- 1/2 cup Epsom salts
- 10 drops lavender essential oil

Directions:

1. Fill a bathtub with warm water.
2. Add castor oil, Epsom salts, and lavender essential oil.
3. Soak for 20-30 minutes to help relax muscles and reduce soreness.

Castor Oil and Cayenne Pepper Heating Salve

Ingredients:

- 2 tablespoons castor oil
- 1 teaspoon cayenne pepper
- 1 tablespoon beeswax pellets

Directions:

1. Heat castor oil and beeswax in a double boiler until the beeswax melts.
2. Stir in cayenne pepper.
3. Pour into a container and let cool. Apply to painful muscles for a warming sensation.

Castor Oil and Ginger Muscle Rub

Ingredients:

- 3 tablespoons castor oil
- 2 teaspoons fresh ginger juice or 1 teaspoon ginger powder

Directions:

1. Mix castor oil with ginger.

2. Massage directly onto sore muscles to help reduce stiffness and soreness.

Castor Oil for Headache and Migraine Relief

Utilize castor oil's soothing properties to alleviate headaches and migraines with these simple remedies.

Castor Oil Scalp Massage

Ingredients:

- 2 tablespoons castor oil
- 5 drops peppermint essential oil

Directions:

1. Mix castor oil with peppermint essential oil.

2. Gently massage into the scalp, focusing on temples and neck.

3. Use at the onset of migraine symptoms for relief.

Castor Oil and Lavender Head Compress

Ingredients:

- Castor oil
- Lavender essential oil
- Warm water

- Soft cloth

Directions:

1. Mix lavender essential oil with castor oil.

2. Soak a cloth in warm water, wring out, and drizzle with oil mixture.

3. Apply as a compress to forehead or neck to reduce symptoms.

Castor Oil Temple Rub

Ingredients:

- Castor oil

- 2 drops eucalyptus oil

Directions:

1. Blend castor oil with eucalyptus oil.

2. Gently rub onto temples and forehead for a calming effect.

Relaxing Castor Oil Bath

Ingredients:

- ¼ cup castor oil

- ½ cup Epsom salts

- 10 drops lavender or chamomile essential oil

Directions:

1. Fill a bath with warm water.

2. Add castor oil, Epsom salts, and essential oil.

3. Soak for 20-30 minutes to relieve migraine symptoms.

Castor Oil Neck Wrap

Ingredients:

- Castor oil

- Hot water bottle or heating pad

- Soft cloth

Directions:

1. Soak a cloth in warm castor oil.

2. Apply around the neck.

3. Cover with a hot water bottle or heating pad to enhance relaxation and pain relief.

Castor Oil and Rosemary Oil Blend

Ingredients:

- 2 tablespoons castor oil

- 3 drops rosemary essential oil

Directions:

1. Mix castor oil with rosemary essential oil.

2. Massage into the scalp around painful areas for migraine relief.

Natural Castor Oil Remedies for Health Issues

Castor Oil for Constipation Relief

Castor oil has long been used as a natural remedy for constipation due to its laxative properties. Below are various methods to incorporate castor oil into treatments for effective relief.

Milk and Castor Oil for Constipation

Ingredients:

- Warm milk: 1 glass
- Castor oil: 1 tablespoon

Directions:

1. Stir the warm milk with the castor oil.
2. Drink the mixture just before bedtime for optimal benefits.

Prunes and Castor Oil for Constipation

Ingredients:

- Dried prunes: 3-4
- Castor oil: 1 tablespoon

Directions:

1. Soak the prunes in water to soften them.
2. Mash the prunes and mix with castor oil. Eat the mixture.

Sweet Potato and Castor Oil for Constipation

Ingredients:

- Boiled sweet potato: 1
- Castor oil: 1 tablespoon

Directions:

1. Mash the boiled sweet potato.

2.   Mix in the castor oil and consume as a nutritious remedy for constipation.

Castor Oil and Heating Pad for Constipation

Ingredients:

*   Heating pad

*   Castor oil: 1 tablespoon

Directions:

1.   Rub castor oil all over your abdomen.

2.   Place the heating pad over the oiled area for 10-15 minutes to enhance oil absorption and relieve discomfort.

Castor Oil and Honey for Constipation

Ingredients:

*   Honey: 1 tablespoon

*   Castor oil: 1 tablespoon

Directions:

1.   Mix the honey and castor oil.

2.   Drink the mixture to alleviate constipation.

Castor Oil and Lemon Juice for Constipation

Ingredients:

*   Lemon juice: half a lemon

*   Castor oil: 1 tablespoon

Directions:

1.   Mix freshly squeezed lemon juice with castor oil and drink.

2.   Optionally, apply this mixture to your stomach to help with absorption.

Castor Oil for Anxiety Relief

Relaxing Castor Oil Scalp Massage

Ingredients:

*   Castor oil: 2 tablespoons

*   Lavender essential oil: 2 drops

Directions:

1.   Mix castor oil with lavender essential oil.

2.   Apply to your scalp and massage gently in circular motions to relieve tension and promote relaxation.

Castor Oil and Chamomile Foot Rub

Ingredients:

*   Castor oil: 3 tablespoons

*   Chamomile essential oil: 3 drops

Directions:

1.   Mix the oils and warm slightly.

2.   Massage into your feet, especially the pressure points, and wear socks to enhance absorption and relaxation.

Calming Castor Oil Bath

Ingredients:

- Castor oil: ¼ cup

- Epsom salts: ½ cup

- Calming essential oil (e.g., rose or sandalwood): 10 drops

Directions:

1. Fill a bathtub with warm water.

2. Add castor oil, Epsom salts, and essential oil.

3. Soak for 20-30 minutes to soothe nerves and relax your body.

Castor Oil Aromatherapy Diffuser Blend

Ingredients:

- Castor oil: 1 tablespoon (as a carrier)

- Bergamot essential oil: 4 drops

- Frankincense essential oil: 2 drops

Directions:

1. Mix the oils in a small bottle.

2. Use a few drops in your diffuser to create a calming atmosphere.

Soothing Castor Oil Compress

Ingredients:

- Castor oil

- Warm water

- Soft cloth

Directions:

1.   Soak a cloth in warm castor oil.

2.   Apply it to the back of your neck or forehead to alleviate anxiety symptoms.

Castor Oil and Peppermint Neck Massage

Ingredients:

- Castor oil: 2 tablespoons

- Peppermint essential oil: 3 drops

Directions:

1.   Mix castor oil with peppermint essential oil.

2.   Warm slightly and massage into your neck and shoulders to relieve stress and anxiety.

Castor Oil for Stress and Wellness Remedies

Soothing Massage Oil

Ingredients:

- Castor oil: 1 tablespoon

- Almond oil: 9 tablespoons

- Essential oils of your choice

Procedure:

1.   Mix castor oil with almond oil in a glass bowl. Add a few drops of your preferred essential oils such as lavender, chamomile, or sandalwood.

2.   Use this blend for full-body massages after a shower or apply to temples, neck, and stomach before sleep.

Benefits: Castor oil is renowned for its anti-inflammatory properties, helping to ease joint pain and muscle aches. It also promotes blood circulation, which supports a healthy lymphatic system. This system helps fight bacteria and disease, enhancing overall health and immune function.

Simple Relaxing Massage Oil

Ingredients:

3 tablespoons castor oil

5-6 drops lavender essential oil

3-4 drops bergamot essential oil

3-4 drops chamomile essential oil

Directions:

Combine all essential oils with castor oil in a small bottle.

Shake well to mix.

To use, warm a few drops between your hands and massage into the shoulders and neck to release tension before sleep.

Castor Oil Stress-Relief Massage Blend

Ingredients:

2 tablespoons castor oil

5 drops lavender essential oil

3 drops chamomile essential oil

Directions:

In a small bottle, mix the castor oil with the lavender and chamomile essential oils.

Gently massage the blend into your temples, neck, and shoulders to help alleviate stress and induce relaxation.

Castor Oil Foot Soak

Ingredients:

¼ cup castor oil

Warm water

A few drops of eucalyptus or peppermint essential oil

Directions:

Fill a foot bath with warm water, then add the castor oil and essential oil.

Soak your feet for 20-30 minutes to help soothe aches and relax.

Castor Oil and Coconut Oil Scalp Massage

Ingredients:

1 tablespoon castor oil

1 tablespoon coconut oil

2 drops rosemary essential oil (optional)

Directions:

Mix the oils in a small bowl.

Slightly warm the mixture.

Use to massage the scalp, helping to relieve tension and enhance relaxation.

Castor Oil Bath Additive

Ingredients:

1/4 cup castor oil

1/2 cup Epsom salts

10 drops calming essential oil (e.g., lavender, frankincense)

Directions:

Blend the castor oil with Epsom salts and essential oil.

Add to a warm bath and soak for at least 20 minutes to relax muscles and soothe stress.

Relaxing Castor Oil Compress

Ingredients:

Castor oil

Warm water

Soft cloth

Directions:

Soak a cloth in warm castor oil.

Apply to the forehead, back of the neck, or lower back.

Cover with a warm towel or heating pad and let sit for about 30 minutes for deep relaxation.

Castor Oil Aromatherapy Diffuser Blend

Ingredients:

1 tablespoon castor oil (as carrier oil)

4 drops bergamot essential oil

2 drops sandalwood essential oil

Directions:

Mix the castor oil with the bergamot and sandalwood essential oils.

Add a few drops to the water reservoir of an oil diffuser.

Run the diffuser to create a relaxing atmosphere in your home or office.

Castor Oil for Gut and Liver Health

Castor Oil Pack for Gut

Ingredients:

Castor oil

Cotton flannel

Plastic wrap

Heating pad or hot water bottle

Directions:

Saturate a piece of cotton flannel with castor oil until thoroughly soaked but not dripping.

Position the flannel over your abdomen.

Cover with plastic wrap to prevent leakage.

Place a heating pad or hot water bottle over the plastic to apply gentle heat.

Leave in place for 1-2 hours to enhance circulation and support detoxification. Perform this 2-3 times a week.

Internal Castor Oil Cleanse

Ingredients:

1 to 2 tablespoons of castor oil

Directions:

Consume castor oil on an empty stomach in the morning; mix with a small amount of juice to improve flavor if necessary.

Stay near a bathroom, as castor oil can act as a potent laxative.

Use this cleanse sparingly to avoid dependency or disruption of normal gut functions.

Castor Oil and Ginger Massage Oil

Ingredients:

2 tablespoons castor oil

1 teaspoon ginger juice or 3 drops ginger essential oil

Directions:

Mix castor oil with ginger juice or ginger essential oil.

Warm the mixture slightly, then gently massage it over your abdomen.

The warming properties of ginger combined with castor oil can stimulate digestion and cleanse the gut. Perform this massage nightly before bed.

Castor Oil Herbal Tea

Ingredients:

1 tablespoon castor oil

1 cup herbal tea (peppermint or chamomile recommended)

Directions:

Brew a cup of herbal tea and let it cool slightly.

Stir in a tablespoon of castor oil.

Drink this tea early in the morning on an empty stomach to help lubricate the intestines and facilitate a gentle cleanse.

Abdominal Castor Oil Compress

Ingredients:

Castor oil

Warm water

Hand towel or small cloth

Directions:

Soak a hand towel or small cloth in warm castor oil.

Wring out excess oil and place the cloth on your abdomen.

Cover with plastic wrap and a heating pad for about 30-45 minutes to enhance absorption and effectiveness. Repeat a few times a week.

Castor Oil and Lemon Detox Wrap

Ingredients:

3 tablespoons castor oil

5 drops lemon essential oil

Directions:

Mix castor oil with lemon essential oil.

Apply the mixture over your abdomen and wrap with a clean bandage or cloth.

Cover with a warm heating pad for about an hour to promote detoxification through the skin. Use once or twice a week.

Standard Castor Oil Pack for Liver

Ingredients:

Castor oil

Cotton flannel

Plastic wrap

Heating pad or hot water bottle

Directions:

Saturate a piece of cotton flannel in castor oil.

Place the flannel over your liver area (right side of the abdomen, just below the rib cage).

Cover with plastic wrap to prevent staining.

Apply a heating pad or hot water bottle for gentle heat.

Keep the pack in place for 45-60 minutes. Repeat 2-3 times a week to assist in liver detoxification.

Detoxifying Castor Oil Massage

Ingredients:

2 tablespoons castor oil

2 drops cypress essential oil (optional)

Directions:

Slightly warm the castor oil and mix with cypress essential oil if using.

Massage the oil mixture over your abdomen, focusing on the liver area.

Perform the massage before bed to allow the oil to work overnight, showering in the morning if desired.

Castor Oil and Lemon Foot Rub

Ingredients:

1 tablespoon castor oil

2 drops lemon essential oil

Directions:

Blend the castor oil with lemon essential oil.

Massage the mixture onto the soles of your feet, concentrating on reflex points linked to the liver.

Cover your feet with socks overnight to enhance absorption. Repeat nightly for a week.

Castor Oil Hot Compress

Ingredients:

Castor oil

Hand towel or small cloth

Directions:

Soak the towel or cloth in warm castor oil.

Apply it directly to the liver area and cover with plastic wrap.

Place a hot water bottle or heating pad over the compress for about 30-45 minutes. Repeat 3 times a week.

Refreshing Castor Oil Bath

Ingredients:

1/4 cup castor oil

1/2 cup Epsom salts

5 drops grapefruit essential oil (optional for additional detoxification support)

Directions:

Fill your bathtub with warm water and add the castor oil, Epsom salts, and grapefruit essential oil.

Soak in the bath for at least 20 minutes to allow your body to detoxify.

Try to relax completely, letting the ingredients work their detoxifying magic. It's recommended to do this once a week for best results.

Liver Support Castor Oil Blend

Ingredients:

3 tablespoons castor oil

2 drops rosemary essential oil

1 drop geranium essential oil

Directions:

Mix the castor oil with rosemary and geranium essential oils. This combination is thought to enhance liver function.

Apply the oil blend to the liver area, which is on the right side of your abdomen, just below the rib cage. Gently massage in a clockwise direction.

Cover the area with a warm cloth or heating pad for about 30 minutes to increase the effectiveness of the oils. Wash off afterward.

Use this treatment 2-3 times per week for optimal liver support.

Natural Castor Oil Women's Health Remedies

Castor Oil for the Vagina

Castor Oil Pack for Pelvic Area

Ingredients:

Castor oil

Cotton flannel

Plastic wrap

Heating pad or hot water bottle

Directions:

Soak a piece of cotton flannel in castor oil until it is fully saturated but not dripping.

Place the flannel on the lower abdomen or pelvic area, avoiding direct contact with the genitals.

Cover with plastic wrap to prevent oil leakage onto clothing or bedding.

Place a heating pad or hot water bottle over the plastic wrap to provide gentle heat.

Maintain this setup for 30-60 minutes. This treatment is beneficial for easing menstrual cramps or pelvic pain.

External Soothing Castor Oil Blend for Itch Relief

Ingredients:

2 tablespoons castor oil

1 tablespoon coconut oil

2 drops lavender essential oil (optional for added soothing properties)

Directions:

Thoroughly mix all ingredients in a clean container.

Apply the mixture externally around the vulva, not internally, particularly if experiencing irritation or dryness.

Use this blend at night since coconut oil can be messy. It offers soothing moisture and potential anti-inflammatory benefits.

Castor Oil Compress for External Use

Ingredients:

Castor oil

Warm water

Soft cloth

Directions:

Soak a small cloth in warm castor oil.

Place the cloth on the external genital area or lower abdomen to alleviate discomfort.

Avoid applying heat and do not use internally. This treatment can be used for 15-20 minutes to reduce discomfort related to conditions like yeast infections or vulvodynia, always consult medical advice.

Gentle Massage Oil for Lower Abdomen

Ingredients:

3 tablespoons castor oil

1 tablespoon jojoba oil

2 drops chamomile essential oil

Directions:

Mix all oils in a small container thoroughly.

Gently massage the oil into the lower abdomen to help soothe menstrual cramps or pelvic pain.

Ensure to apply it only to the lower abdomen, not directly to the genital area.

Soothing Bath Additive

Ingredients:

¼ cup castor oil

½ cup Epsom salts

A few drops of chamomile or lavender essential oil for additional relaxation

Directions:

Fill your bathtub with warm water and add the Epsom salts and castor oil.

Incorporate a few drops of chamomile or lavender essential oil.

Soak in the tub for 20-30 minutes, focusing on relaxing the pelvic muscles. This can help relieve cramps and calm nerves.

Hydrating and Soothing External Rub

Ingredients:

2 tablespoons castor oil

1 tablespoon aloe vera gel

1 teaspoon vitamin E oil

Directions:

Combine castor oil, aloe vera gel, and vitamin E oil in a bowl.

Apply the mixture externally around the vulva to hydrate and soothe the area.

This rub is particularly beneficial if experiencing dryness or irritation in the vulvar area.

Castor Oil for Hormones

Castor Oil Pack for Hormonal Balance

Ingredients:

- Castor oil

- Cotton flannel

- Plastic wrap

- Heating pad or hot water bottle

Directions:

1. Soak cotton flannel in castor oil.

2. Place over lower abdomen.

3. Cover with plastic wrap; apply heat for 30-60 minutes, 2-3 times weekly.

Castor Oil and Clary Sage Massage Oil

Ingredients:

- 2 tablespoons castor oil

- 5 drops clary sage essential oil

Directions:

1. Mix castor oil with clary sage essential oil.

2. Massage onto abdomen, lower back, and discomfort areas during menstrual cycle.

3. Clary sage may help balance estrogen levels and relieve menstrual pain.

Evening Primrose and Castor Oil Blend

Ingredients:

- 1 tablespoon castor oil
- 1 tablespoon evening primrose oil

Directions:

1. Combine oils in a bottle.

2. Apply to skin, massaging gently on neck, shoulders, and abdomen.

3. Evening primrose oil, known for hormonal health, can be enhanced when combined with castor oil.

Midwife Brew Recipe

Ingredients:

- 10 oz apricot juice
- 8 oz lemon verbena tea
- 2 tbsp castor oil
- 2 tbsp almond butter

Directions:

1. Brew lemon verbena tea in boiling water for at least 10 minutes.

2. Blend all ingredients until smooth.

3. Consume on empty stomach.

Castor Oil Scalp Treatment for Thyroid Health

Ingredients:

- 2 tablespoons castor oil

- 2 drops rosemary essential oil

Directions:

1. Blend castor oil with rosemary essential oil.

2. Massage into scalp to potentially support thyroid function.

3. Repeat several times a week, especially before showering.

Soothing Castor Oil

Bath Ingredients:

- ¼ cup castor oil

- ¼ cup Epsom salts

- 10 drops lavender essential oil

Directions:

1. Fill bathtub with warm water; add castor oil, Epsom salts, and lavender essential oil.

2. Soak for 20-30 minutes to relax body and support hormonal health.

3. Ideal before bedtime for improved sleep quality.

Castor Oil Foot Rub for Endocrine Support

Ingredients:

- 2 tablespoons castor oil

- 3 drops geranium essential oil

Directions:

1. Mix castor oil with geranium essential oil.

2. Massage into feet, focusing on reflexology points linked to endocrine glands.

3. Wear socks overnight for deep absorption.

Castor Oil for Menstrual Pain

Basic Castor Oil Pack

Ingredients:

- Castor oil
- Soft cloth or flannel
- Plastic wrap
- Heating pad or hot water bottle

Directions:

1. Soak cloth in castor oil.

2. Place on lower abdomen.

3. Cover with plastic wrap; apply heat for 30-60 minutes.

Castor Oil and Lavender Massage

Ingredients:

- ¼ cup castor oil
- 5-7 drops lavender essential oil

Directions:

1.   Mix castor oil with lavender essential oil.

2.   Warm slightly; massage onto lower abdomen in circular motions for pain relief.

Herbal Castor Oil Blend

Ingredients:

- ¼ cup castor oil
- 5 drops clary sage essential oil
- 5 drops peppermint essential oil

Directions:

1.   Combine oils; apply generously to lower abdomen.

2.   Cover with warm cloth or heating pad for absorption and pain relief.

Soothing Castor Oil Bath

Ingredients:

- ¼ cup castor oil
- ½ cup Epsom salts
- 10 drops essential oil (e.g., rose or chamomile)

Directions:

1.   Fill bathtub with warm water.

2.   Add castor oil, Epsom salts, and essential oils; soak for 20 minutes.

3.   Relaxes muscles and eases menstrual pain.

Castor Oil Hot Compress

Ingredients:

- Castor oil

- Small towel or handkerchief

Directions:

1. Warm castor oil.

2. Soak towel; apply to lower abdomen.

3. Cover with plastic; use heating pad for 30 minutes for relief.

Aromatic Castor Oil Compress

Ingredients:

- ¼ cup castor oil

- ¼ cup coconut oil

- 5 drops jasmine essential oil

Directions:

1. Combine castor oil, coconut oil, and jasmine essential oil.

2. Soak a cloth in the oil mixture.

3. Apply to abdomen, cover with plastic wrap, and place warm compress or heating pad over it.

4. Leave for 30 minutes to ease discomfort.

Castor Oil for Infection

Castor Oil Skin Antiseptic

Ingredients:

- 2 tablespoons castor oil
- 3-4 drops tea tree oil

Directions:

1. Mix castor oil with tea tree oil.
2. Clean affected area; apply oil mixture with cotton ball or fingertips.
3. Cover with bandage if needed. Repeat 2-3 times daily.

Castor Oil and Turmeric

Paste Ingredients:

- 1 tablespoon castor oil
- 1 teaspoon turmeric powder

Directions:

1. Combine castor oil and turmeric powder to form paste.
2. Apply directly to infected area.
3. Cover with bandage; leave for few hours or overnight.
4. Rinse off with warm water. Repeat daily.

Castor Oil Wound Salve

Ingredients:

- 2 tablespoons castor oil
- 1 tablespoon coconut oil
- 2-3 drops lavender essential oil (optional)

Directions:

1. Gently heat coconut oil until melted; mix with castor oil.

2. Add lavender essential oil; stir.

3. Apply to clean wound; cover with cloth or bandage. Reapply 2 times daily.

Castor Oil and Garlic Ear Drops

Ingredients:

- 2 tablespoons castor oil
- 1 clove garlic, crushed

Directions:

1. Warm castor oil; add crushed garlic.

2. Infuse for 1-2 hours; strain garlic.

3. Apply 2-3 drops into affected ear once daily for minor infections.

Castor Oil Soothing Compress

Ingredients:

- ¼ cup castor oil
- Warm water

Directions:

1. Soak cloth in warm castor oil.

2. Apply to affected area; cover with plastic wrap.

3. Place heating pad over it; leave for 30-60 minutes. Repeat daily.

Castor Oil and Eucalyptus Respiratory Rub

Ingredients:

- 2 tablespoons castor oil
- 3-4 drops eucalyptus essential oil

Directions:

1. Mix castor oil with eucalyptus oil.

2. Rub onto chest to clear nasal passages and relieve respiratory symptoms.

3. Use before sleep for nighttime relief.

Natural Castor Oil Recipes for Making Soaps and Candles

Candle:

Enhanced Scent Throw Candle

Ingredients:

- 1 cup soy wax flakes
- 1 tablespoon castor oil
- 30 drops essential oil
- Candle wick

Directions:

1. Melt soy wax; stir in castor oil.
2. Add essential oil; mix.
3. Pour into mold; set wick. Let cool and solidify.

Massage Candle

Ingredients:

- ½ cup soy wax
- ¼ cup shea butter
- ¼ cup castor oil
- Essential oils

Directions:

1. Melt soy wax and shea butter; mix in castor oil and essential oils.

2.   Pour into container; let cool. Use as warm massage oil.

Castor Oil Citronella Candle for Outdoors

Ingredients:

- 1 cup paraffin wax
- 2 tablespoons castor oil
- Citronella oil
- Wick, outdoor container

Directions:

1.   Melt paraffin wax; stir in castor oil and citronella oil.
2.   Pour into container; set wick. Let solidify. Use outdoors.

Holiday Spice Candle

Ingredients:

- 1 cup beeswax
- 2 tablespoons castor oil
- Holiday spice essential oils
- Wick, mold

Directions:

1.   Melt beeswax; mix in castor oil and spice oils.
2.   Pour into mold; set wick. Let cool.

Relaxing Lavender Candle

Ingredients:

- 1 cup soy wax
- 1 tablespoon castor oil
- Lavender essential oil
- Wick, container

Directions:

1. Melt soy wax; stir in castor oil and lavender oil.
2. Pour into container; set wick. Let solidify.

Vanilla Bean Coffee Candle

Ingredients:

- 1 cup soy wax
- 1 tablespoon castor oil
- Vanilla essential oil
- Coffee beans
- Wick, container

Directions:

1. Melt soy wax; stir in castor oil and vanilla oil.
2. Place coffee beans in container; pour wax over them. Set wick; let cool.

Peppermint Eucalyptus Energizing Candle

Ingredients:

- 1 cup soy wax
- 1 tablespoon castor oil
- Peppermint and eucalyptus essential oils
- Wick, mold Directions:
1. Melt wax; mix in castor oil and essential oils.
2. Pour into mold; set wick. Let set.

Sea Breeze Candle

Ingredients:

- 1 cup soy wax
- 1 tablespoon castor oil
- Sea breeze fragrance oil
- Wick, container

Directions:

1. Melt wax; mix in castor oil and fragrance oil.
2. Pour into container; set wick. Let solidify.

Massage Oil Candle

Prep Time: 10 minutes

Cook Time: 20 minutes

Total Time: 30 minutes

Servings: 1 candle (2.5 ounces)

Equipment:

- Heat Safe Container
- Pan for boiling water
- Spatula
- Scale
- Marker (to hold wick straight)
- Scissors
- Glue gun
- Candle Container

Ingredients:

- 0.70-ounce Soy Wax (28%)
- 0.78-ounce Cocoa Butter Deodorized (31%)
- 0.80-ounce Shea Butter Refined (32%)
- 0.13-ounce Caster Oil (5%)
- 0.10-ounce Love Spell Fragrance Oil (4%) **Follow manufacturer's recommendation for use rate
- 1 Wick
- 1 Candle Container

Instructions:

1. Adhere the wick to the candle jar's bottom using a small amount of hot glue.

2. Ensure the wick is centered in the jar.

3. Weigh all ingredients.

4. **Heated Phase:**

- Add soy wax and cocoa butter to your heat-safe container.

- Place in a double boiler until fully melted, stirring to avoid overheating.

5.   **Cool Down Phase:**

- Add shea butter, melting it into the mixture.

- Stir in castor oil and fragrance oil.

- Mix thoroughly.

- Pour into the candle container.

- Use a marker to keep the wick centered as it cools.

- Allow the candle to cool completely.

- Trim the wick to 1/4 inch.

Soap:

Goat's Milk and Lavender Melt and Pour Shampoo Bar

Ingredients:

- 1 lb. Organic Goat's Milk Glycerin Melt & Pour Soap Base

- 1 tsp Mango Butter

- 2 tsp Castor Oil

- 20 – 25 drops of high-quality lavender essential oil

Instructions:

1.   Cut the soap base and gently melt on low heat.

2.   Add mango butter, letting it melt.

3.   Remove from heat; stir in castor oil and lavender oil.

4.   Ensure the mold is on a level surface; pour the mixture nearly level.

5.   Spray with rubbing alcohol to prevent air bubbles.

6.   Let cool for several hours.

7.   Gently remove from the mold.

8.   Store in an air-tight container for up to a year.

How to Use: Wet hair, then wet the shampoo bar. Create a lather in your hands or apply directly to your scalp and hair. Rinse well.

Beeswax Citrus Soap Recipe

Equipment:

- Immersion blender
- Digital cooking thermometer
- Kitchen scale
- Variety of containers and pots for soap making
- Soap mold (e.g., small kitty litter pan or milk container)
- Old clothes and apron
- Goggles
- Rubber Gloves

Ingredients:

- 36 ounces olive oil
- 6 ounces coconut oil
- 3 ounces castor oil
- 2 ounces grated beeswax
- 12 ounces distilled water
- 6 ounces lye
- 2 ounces essential oil (e.g., Vitamin E and orange oil)

Instructions:

1.   Measure 12 ounces of water into a plastic pitcher, set in the sink.

2.   Weigh 6 ounces of lye in a plastic cup.

3.   Carefully add lye to the water, stirring gently. It will heat up and emit fumes.

4.   Set the pitcher outside to cool.

5.   Weigh and heat oils and beeswax until dissolved.

6.   Allow the oil mixture to cool to about 98 to 110 degrees F.

7.   Ensure the lye solution cools to a similar temperature.

8.   Prepare the immersion blender.

9.   Pour the lye solution into the oil mixture, stirring manually before blending.

10.   Blend until the mixture reaches "trace" (consistency of runny pudding).

11.   Add essential oils and optional grated orange peel and turmeric for color.

12.   Pour into the mold, cover with an old towel, and set aside for 24 hours.

13.   Cut into blocks the next day.

This batch can produce 20 blocks of soap, ideal for personal use and as gifts.

Cold Process Soap Recipe

This recipe yields eight bars of soap, but it can be halved or quartered for smaller batches.

Ingredients:

- 63g Sodium Hydroxide (Lye)

- 113g Distilled Water

- 114g Fractionated Coconut Oil

- 91g Shea Butter

- 227g Light Colored Olive Oil

- 23g Castor Oil

- Essential Oils (1-3% of the total recipe, adjust based on potency)

Adding Essential Oils:

- Gentle oils like Mandarin: Up to 20g (about 3%)

- Potent oils like Cinnamon: Up to 7g (about 1%)

- Blend example: 13g Mandarin with 7g Cinnamon

Method:

1.   Dissolve sodium hydroxide in water by pouring lye into the water (never reverse), then set aside.

2.   Melt coconut oil and shea butter gently, remove from heat once melted.

3.   In a separate container, combine olive oil, castor oil, and essential oils.

4.   Allow the oil mix to cool to 35-38°C. Ensure the lye water is at a similar temperature.

5.   Slowly pour the lye water through a sieve into the oil mix.

6.   Stir well, then blend with a stick blender in short bursts until reaching 'trace' (thin, custard-like consistency).

7.   Quickly pour into a mold, tap to settle.

8.   For quick results, refrigerate overnight. After 48 hours, unmold and cut into bars.

9.   Soap can be used now but curing for 28 days in a cool, dry place improves quality and longevity.

10.   For a hot process variation, heat the mixture in a crock pot during step 6 until it reaches a Vaseline-like consistency, then mold.

Gentle Cold Process Soap with Shea Butter

Ingredients:

- 400g Extra Virgin Olive Oil
- 75g Organic Unrefined Shea Butter (or refined if preferred)
- 25g Castor Oil
- 130g Distilled Water
- 63.62g Sodium Hydroxide (Lye)

Instructions:

1. Wear protective gear. Measure water into a stainless-steel container.
2. Separately measure the lye.
3. Slowly add lye to water, stir until clear, and set aside to cool.
4. Measure oils and butter, heat gently to 38-42°C.
5. Combine lye solution with oils/butter, mix to trace.
6. Pour into a mold, let set for 24-48 hours.
7. After hardening, unmold and cut into bars.
8. Cure bars on a rack for 6-8 weeks before use.

Basic Castor Oil Soap

Ingredients:

- 6 oz. Coconut Oil
- 6 oz. Olive Oil
- 2 oz. Castor Oil
- 2.2 oz. Lye (Sodium Hydroxide)
- 6 oz. Water

Directions:

1. Mix lye into water and cool.

2. Melt coconut oil, blend with olive and castor oils.

3. Add lye water to oils, blend to trace.

4. Pour into a mold, cover, and insulate for 24 hours.

5. Unmold, cut into bars, and cure for 4-6 weeks.

Lavender Castor Soap

Ingredients:

- 4 oz. castor oil

- 10 oz. olive oil

- 6 oz. coconut oil

- 2 oz. shea butter

- 4.3 oz. lye (sodium hydroxide)

- 10 oz. water

- 1 oz. lavender essential oil

Directions:

1. Carefully mix the lye into the water and set it aside to cool.

2. Melt the coconut oil and shea butter, then add the olive and castor oils.

3. Once the lye water and oils are cool, combine and blend until the mixture reaches trace.

4. Add lavender essential oil, stir thoroughly, and pour into molds.

5. Allow the soap to cure as described in the basic method above.

Honey and Oatmeal Castor Soap

Ingredients:

- 2 oz. castor oil
- 8 oz. coconut oil
- 8 oz. olive oil
- 1 oz. raw honey
- 1 oz. ground oatmeal
- 3.2 oz. lye
- 8 oz. water

Directions:

1. Mix the lye into the water and allow to cool.

2. Melt the coconut oil, then blend in the olive and castor oils.

3. Once the lye water and oils are combined at trace, stir in honey and ground oatmeal.

4. Pour into molds and allow to cure as described above.

Peppermint Castor Soap

Ingredients:

- 2 oz. castor oil
- 10 oz. palm oil
- 6 oz. coconut oil
- 4 oz. olive oil
- 4.5 oz. lye
- 8 oz. water
- 1 oz. peppermint essential oil

Directions:

1.   Prepare the lye water and let it cool.

2.   Melt the palm and coconut oils, then add the olive and castor oils.

3.   Combine the lye water with the oils once they reach trace, then add the peppermint oil and mix thoroughly.

4.   Pour into molds and allow to cure as previously described.

Lemon Zest Castor Soap

Ingredients:

- 2 oz. castor oil
- 8 oz. coconut oil
- 8 oz. olive oil
- 1 tbsp lemon zest
- 3.2 oz. lye
- 8 oz. water

Directions:

1.   Prepare the lye water and allow it to cool.

2.   Melt the coconut oil and blend with the olive and castor oils.

3.   Once at trace, add lemon zest and mix thoroughly.

4.   Pour into molds and cure as outlined above.

Coffee Grounds Exfoliating Soap

Ingredients:

- 2 oz. castor oil
- 6 oz. olive oil
- 6 oz. coconut oil
- 2 oz. ground coffee
- 2.2 oz. lye
- 6 oz. water

Directions:

1. Mix the lye into the water and allow it to cool.
2. Melt the coconut oil, then blend in the olive and castor oils.
3. At trace, add the coffee grounds and mix thoroughly.
4. Pour into molds and cure as described above.

Activated Charcoal Detox Soap

Ingredients:

- 2 oz. castor oil
- 8 oz. olive oil
- 8 oz. coconut oil
- 1 oz. activated charcoal
- 3.2 oz. lye
- 8 oz. water

Directions:

1. Prepare the lye solution and allow it to cool.
2. Melt the coconut oil, then blend in the olive and castor oils.
3. At trace, thoroughly mix in the activated charcoal.
4. Pour into molds and allow to cure as outlined above.

References

1.   Achebe, H.O., & Job, I.K. (2020). The therapeutic efficacy of castor oil: An overview of its properties and applications. Journal of Herbal Medicine and Toxicology, 14(2), 33-42. This article provides a comprehensive review of the medicinal properties and historical uses of castor oil.

2.   Brown, M.T. (2018). Castor oil: The natural solution for your beauty needs. Green Beauty Publications. This book offers insights into the practical

uses of castor oil in everyday beauty regimes, detailing recipes and applications for natural skincare.

3.   Dawson, E.K., & Rodriguez, L. (2019). Natural remedies for modern ailments. Holistic Health Press. Chapter 7, "Castor Oil for Digestive Wellness," explores the role of castor oil as a natural laxative and its benefits for digestive health.

4.   National Institute of Health (NIH). (2021). Castor oil. Retrieved from https://www.nih.gov/castor-oil This government health portal provides scientifically-backed data on the nutritional content and safety considerations of using castor oil.

5.   Peters, R. (2017). Essential Oils for Beginners: The Guide to Get Started with Essential Oils and Aromatherapy. New York: Althea Press. Section on castor oil, pp. 145-150, discusses various essential oils, including detailed coverage on castor oil, its extraction processes, and safety tips.

6.   Woods, G. (2022). Unlocking Nature's Secrets: The Ultimate Guide to Natural Remedies. Nature Cure Publishing. This guide includes a detailed chapter on castor oil, highlighting its applications in natural medicine and home remedies.

7.   Green, S. (2023). Nature's Pharmacy: A Comprehensive Guide to Natural Remedies. Wellness Press. This resource explores natural remedies for common ailments and includes an in-depth section on castor oil, its properties, and how it can be used effectively for health and beauty.

8.   Johnson, T. (2021). Encyclopedia of Herbal Medicine. 3rd Edition. DK Publishing. Provides detailed information on various herbs and oils, including castor oil, with a focus on its historical and modern medical applications.

9.   Singh, P., & Kapoor, I.P.S. (2022). Castor Oil as a Bioactive Ingredient: Extraction, Efficacy, and Applications. International Journal of Bioactive Compounds, 8(1), 58-75. This peer-reviewed article details the extraction methods of castor oil and evaluates its efficacy and applications in the pharmaceutical industry.

10.   Martin, A. (2022). Holistic Healing: The Science of Herbal Medicine. Plant Power Press. Chapter 12 focuses on the role of castor oil in traditional and contemporary herbal medicine practices.

11.   Patel, V.R., & Thaker, V.T. (2020). Castor oil: properties, uses, and optimization of processing parameters in commercial production. Lipid Technology, 32(3), 65-72. This article provides an overview of the commercial production process of castor oil and discusses how its properties can be optimized for various uses.

Online Resources

•   Castor Oil Uses and Benefits - Aroma Web

•   This webpage provides an extensive look at the uses and benefits of castor oil in aromatherapy and personal care.

•   WebMD: Castor Oil - WebMD

•   WebMD offers a medically reviewed article on the uses, side effects, interactions, and dosage of castor oil, helping readers make informed health decisions.

•   MedlinePlus: Castor Oil - MedlinePlus

•   This resource from the U.S. National Library of Medicine provides reliable information on castor oil, including its use as a laxative and other medicinal property.

•   Science Direct: Castor Oil - ScienceDirect

•   Science Direct offers a collection of scientific articles and book chapters discussing the chemical properties and industrial applications of castor oil.

•   The Castor Oil Association - Castor Oil Industry Association

•   An industry website that provides information about the production, standards, and uses of castor oil in various industries, including health and beauty.